Tracey Cox

Secrets of a Supersexpert

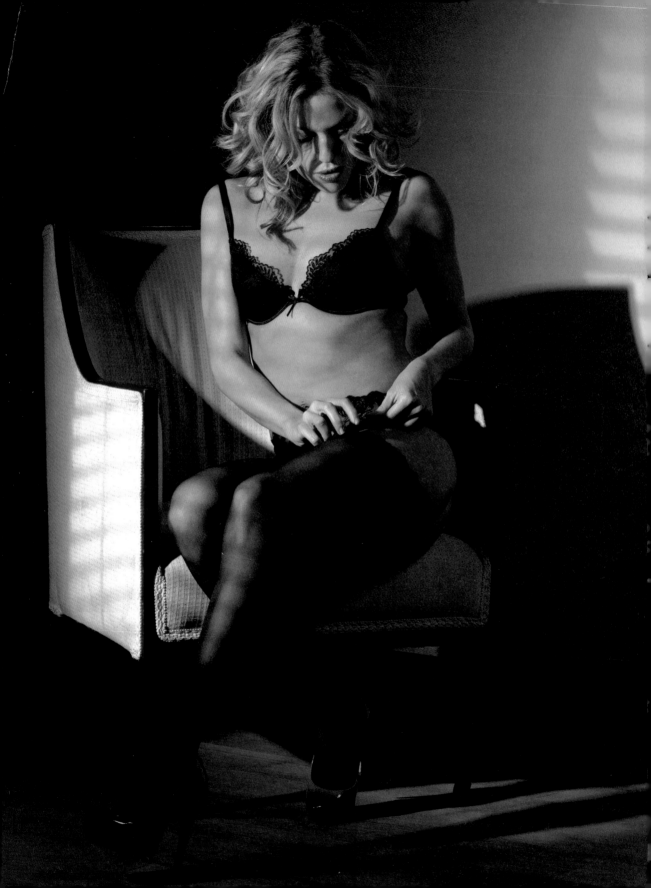

Tracey Cox

Secrets of a Supersexpert

London, New York, Munich, Melbourne, Delhi

Design SEA
Editor Dawn Bates
Senior Art Editor Helen Spencer
Senior Editor Peter Jones
Senior Production Editor Jenny Woodcock
Senior Production Controller Mandy Innes
Managing Art Editor Kat Mead
Executive Managing Editor Adèle Hayward
Art Director Peter Luff
Publisher Stephanie Jackson
US Editor Chuck Wills

Photography Andrew G. Hobbs, John Ross

First American Edition, 2009
Published in the United States by
DK Publishing
375 Hudson Street,
New York, New York 10014

09 10 11 10 9 8 7 6 5 4 3 2 1
SD402—January 2009

Published in Great Britain by Dorling Kindersley Limited.

A catalog record for this book is available from the Library of Congress.

ISBN 978-0-7566-4459-8

DK books are available at special discounts when purchased in bulk for sales promotions, premiums, fund-raising, or educational use. For details, contact: DK Publishing Special Markets, 375 Hudson Street, New York, New York 10014 or SpecialSales@dk.com

Printed in Germany by Mohn Media

Discover more at **www.dk.com**

Neither the publisher nor the author is engaged in rendering professional advice or services to the individual reader, and neither shall be liable or responsible for any loss or damage allegedly rising from any information or suggestion in this book. Anyone participating in the activities that this book discusses or suggests assumes responsibility for his or her own actions and safety, and for compliance with all applicable laws. If you have any health problems or medical conditions, or any other concerns about whether you are able to participate in any of these activities, you should take appropriate precautions. The information contained in this book cannot replace professional advice, or sound judgment and good decision making.

Contents

Chapter One: Getting It

Why you shouldn't always listen to sexperts, boning up on his precious part, keeping up with the Joneses in the bedroom, and why we all have sex on the brain.

Chapter Two: Doing It

How to give and get great oral sex, sinful sex tricks and killer combos, more and better orgasms; and why the G-spot still fascinates.

Chapter Three: Living It

Fix your sex life tonight, what to do if you can't have an orgasm, what he needs to know to be the best she's ever had, and how she can blow his … brain.

Chapter Four: Pushing It

How a butterfly, rabbit, or duck can help pep up your sex life, surviving a threesome, loving porn, tackling net sex, talking dirty, and how to simply talk about sex.

Chapter Five: Believing It

The solutions to some rather undignified sex situations and why a virgin can start fires and catch salmon with her bare hands. Yes, really.

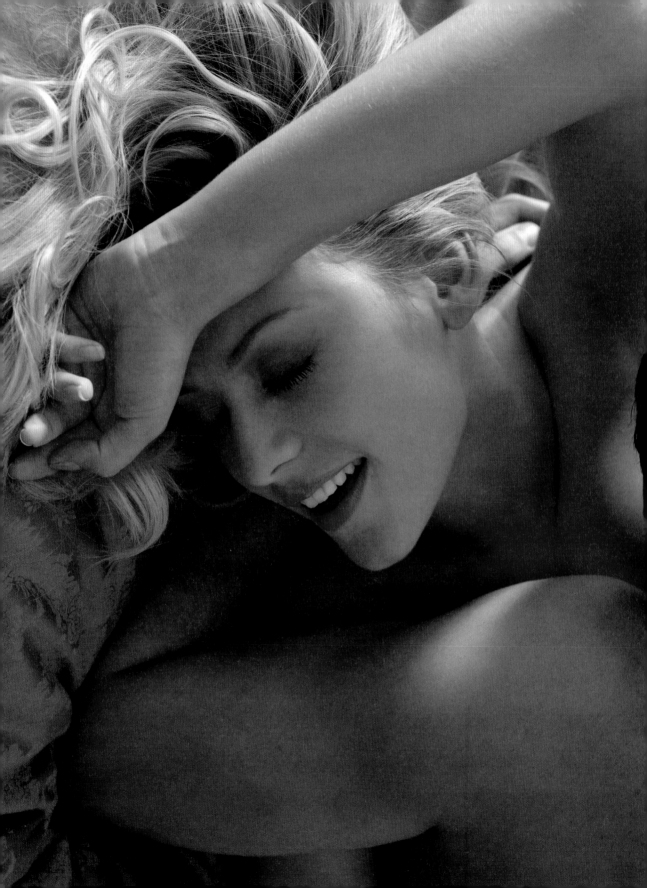

Introduction

It's quite interesting having sex as your speciality topic—you get to know stuff the average person doesn't about the world's all-time favorite obsession. Quite apart from sex being the focus of my professional life—I write books, magazine articles, and do TV and radio shows on the topic worldwide—people tell me things.

Because I'm a sexpert, people have the urge to confess to me. They think I've got the answers—or they think I'm unshockable and simply want to boast. People write to my website, stop me in lines at airports, outside (sometimes inside) the bathrooms at parties, in bars and restaurants, and once in the vegetable section of a supermarket while I was still in my gym clothes and holding a bunch of carrots. People talk—and I listen.

I'm also observant. I read over people's shoulders on planes to see the erotic book hidden inside the novel they're supposedly reading. I peek into women's handbags to see portable vibrators, handcuffs, curious packets of condoms—curious because she's married and I know her husband's had a vasectomy. I watch seemingly loved-up couples at the movies to see who averts their eyes during the sex scenes for hints on which one's in lust, which one's in love. I know that a hand placed on a bottom means a couple are far more likely to be at it than a friendly but asexual arm slung around the waist. I hear stories from people on planes,

after six glasses of wine, and senior citizens on trains, sharp and sober, who lean over to share what they consider are the secrets of a good sex life over sixty.

What do I do with all this information? I keep my mouth shut for starters—if I blabbed, people would stop confiding in me and where's the fun in that? But I keep my mind open, constantly revising how this impacts on how I think about sex and how I'm advising people in my books and TV shows. Am I still on the right track? Are there things I should be covering that I'm not? Am I leading people toward the bedroom for truly satisfying sex or up the garden path? "What's myth, what's reality?" is a question that continually hovers because there's so much nonsense written about sex, it really is hard to separate the two.

This book is the result of more than 15 years solid study, research, and personal reflection on a subject that still fascinates all of us. It's what I thought then, what I know now—and what you can do with this information to make your sex life better than it's ever been. As per usual, I've tried to make the book useful for singles, couples of all ages and stages, and those who are straight, gay, or bi. Please excuse me for mainly using heterosexual references, but it gets a bit complicated trying to cater for all possible combinations. I also want to make it clear everything I suggest assumes you are either practicing safe sex or are in a monogamous relationship where both of you have been tested. There! Now all the formal stuff's out the way, please enjoy! I hope you get as much pleasure reading this as I did writing it!

Tracey

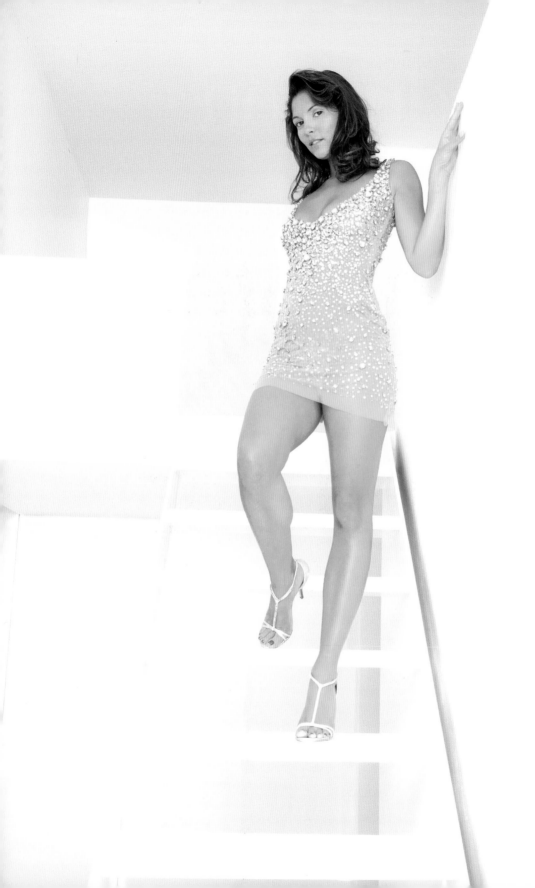

Chapter One

Getting It

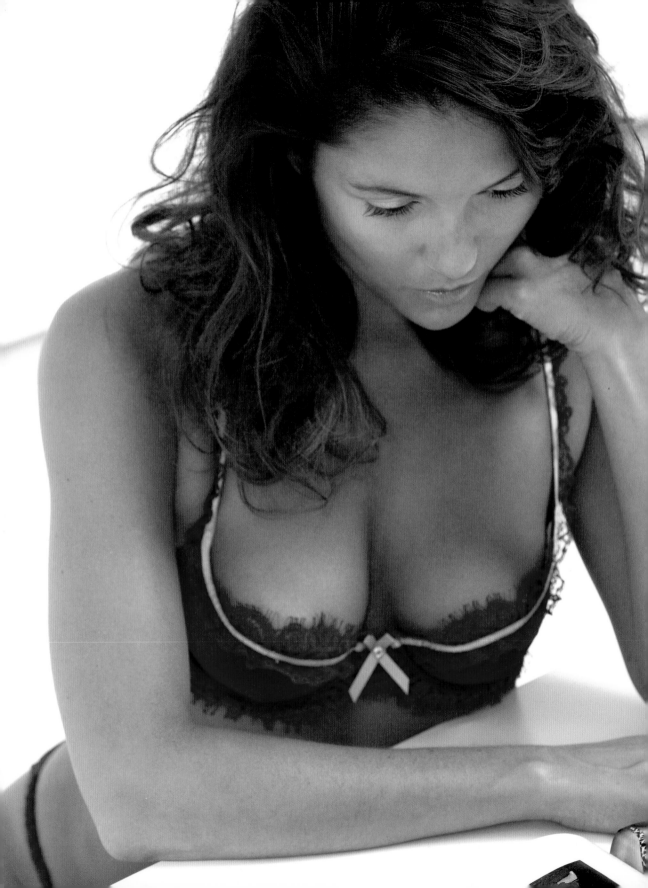

Sex Advice: Is It All A Lot Of Nonsense?

We're told the same stuff over and over—but does the advice us sex experts dole out actually work? New research means some tried-and-tested theories are now done-and-dusted. Here's the lowdown ...

I've written a lot of sex books over the years and given a lot of advice to people. Most of it, I'm proud to say, I still stand by 15 years on. But there's been a plethora of research into arousal and orgasm since I started out as a fledgling "sexpert," and we understand more about our sexual systems and responses now than we ever have. This means the original theories need to be reconsidered—and maybe completely rethought. Some, it has to be said, I will be more than happy to bid farewell to. (I never was fond of the one that said we all had to dress up as doctors and nurses.)

Because we're all individual in our tastes and desires, there has never really been a "this works for everyone" solution to any sexual problem. But there are some pieces of advice doled out by the so-called authorities over and over again. The question is: what's stood the test of time and what's actually a lot of nonsense?

You should talk about sex

It's interesting that no one baulks at taking this advice when their sex life is good; it's only when it's bad that people object to it. In the beginning, you can't shut up about sex—if you're not talking about what you're getting up to already, you're talking about what you'd like to do.

Until something goes wrong. Then it's not quite so much fun because you're feeling a bit delicate after *that* happened, or maybe your partner is, so you sort of shy away from the topic. And just when you really need to be talking about sex—when there's a problem—you both suddenly clam up. Sex then becomes the elephant in the room ... and, more often than not, you both then watch your sex life slide effortlessly down the drain. Here's the deal: no one skates through life without any sex problems and if you can't talk about them, you've got zero chance of solving them. This one is 100 percent accurate, so if you have problems opening up to your partner, turn to pages 146–153 now!

You should plan sex sessions

Advice columnists and "sexperts" often suggest couples book in "date nights" or "sex nights." Now, I'm all for planning—but I do think it has to be done in a certain way or it just becomes another chore added to the list. Instead of planning a "date night," plan an "us" night: a night where just the two of you hang out and do something nice. "Nice" might mean a romantic dinner out, playing a game of tennis together, or simply sitting on the patio with a glass of wine and without the kids.

As for planning sex sessions, again, it really *is* a good idea but it's got to be done with a healthy helping of anticipation or it will work against you. Simply saying, "We've got to have sex tonight" is about as sexy as saying, "Tonight we're going to clean out the closet." But if tonight is the night you're going to try doing something naughty, like tying each other up, spanking each other, visiting a lap-dancing club, suddenly it is exciting. Planning something new and naughty is erotic. Adding sex to the "To Do" list isn't.

You should have sex for 20 minutes or longer

This one came into its own because of a survey that found most women take up to 20 minutes to climax. While everyone took that to mean 20 minutes of general foreplay, it actually meant 20 minutes of direct and consistent clitoral stimulation. So unless the session actually starts with him diving straight for her crown jewel and is over the second she's had her orgasm, it doesn't make sense. People also missed the crucial words "up to," as in it can take women *up to* 20 minutes, rather than it always does. Lots of women are able to orgasm in two minutes, others may take 40 minutes if they're not really in the mood.

Setting a minimum time limit on sex actually damages people's sex lives. If you're struggling to find the energy to even kiss your partner because you're juggling two young kids, trying to hold down a job, and are generally exhausted, being told sex isn't even worth doing unless you're prepared to devote half an hour that you don't have puts lots of couples off doing it at all. The best results I've ever got with couples who'd stopped having sex or had mismatched libidos was to tell them to ignore this piece of advice and instead do the opposite and have sex for no longer than five minutes, three times a week. *Strictly* no longer than five minutes. Now, even the most frazzled or uninterested can cope with a commitment of 15 minutes a week and the person who's desperate for sex at least gets it three times a week. Both are happy, I sit back and wait and, without fail, the next time I see the couple they're grinning from ear to ear. The first thing they confess to is that they were "naughty" and went over the time limit. Of course they did, we always do exactly the opposite to what we're told. Two things work to restore a couple's sexual appetite: remove the pressure and get them having sex again. This technique, sneakily and effectively, does both.

You should roleplay to spice things up

There are those who love dressing up and acting out sexual scenarios and those who would rather strip for their mother-in-law (one who *doesn't* look like Mrs. Robinson). It's one person's idea of heaven, another's hell. As a general rule, I'd say people who like being the center of attention, are unselfconscious, and dream of being "discovered" respond perkily to the suggestion of playing cops and robbers or doctors and nurses. Shy, body-conscious, reserved types simply go pale.

You can judge your relationship by your sex life

It's a good indicator but not a blanket rule. For instance, you'll often have your most intense sex with people who treat you badly. Sex fueled by anxiety, vulnerability, high emotion, and longing for someone we're worried doesn't want us, is drenched with adrenaline. This sharpens nerve endings and makes everything feel way more concentrated. Not all good sex is healthy sex. Couples who argue constantly and feel a lot of anger toward each other often have more explosive sex than couples who get on well and have a good relationship.

In fact, recent research suggests you choose between a great sex life and great relationship! As I hinted at earlier, depressing new evidence suggests the better your relationship, the worse your sex life (but don't give up just yet, there's plenty you can do to fix this on page 112). Statistics also suggest sex accounts for about a quarter of the enjoyment of a relationship, if it's good sex and you're having it regularly. If your sex life is dead or dire, it has a nasty habit of poisoning the rest of your relationship.

You can tell if she's faking it

Men got very excited about the news that a red rash appeared briefly on her chest or neck during an orgasm. At last, a way to tell who's fibbing and who's not! Trouble is, while most people do get the rash, it's not universal so therefore not absolutely reliable. A flushed face, the rash, vaginal contractions, a rapid heart rate, and a clitoris that's sensitive to touch directly afterward are all clues she's genuinely climaxed. But if you want a more accurate assessment than that, you'll need to fork out a couple of million for a device that measures activity in the cerebral cortex. It does exist but whether it would fit comfortably into the bedroom, and be more exciting than a private jet, is questionable. Here's the best way to guarantee your current or next girlfriend won't fake

Danger is what keeps sex red hot long term—this is why couples that are really close friends have problems sustaining desire over time.

it: make it abundantly clear it won't be an issue if she doesn't orgasm. But not in a "I know it's really difficult for women … so let's not even try" type of way. Give us lots of (good) oral sex that lasts a while. Touch us expertly with (lubed-up) fingers. Show just how comfortable you are with yourself by being the one to suggest using a vibrator during intercourse. Then shut up for a while. Nothing worse than being on the brink and you choosing that moment to pop back up, looking expectant, to ask, "Do you think it's going to happen soon?"

Can new underwear really sort your sex problems? Well … yes!

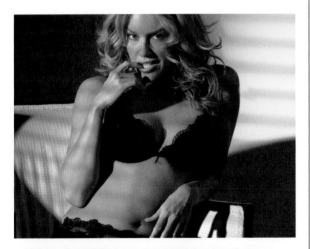

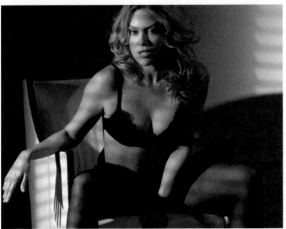

Why she should invest in sexy lingerie

There's always been a perception that all you need to really do to rescue a dire sex life is to pop down to Victoria's Secret and get her to stock up on silk stockings, sheer panties, and boost-up bras. But can new underwear really solve your sex problems? Well … yes! It's not going to solve the serious stuff but if you've just fallen into the been-together-forever rut, it can help because it shows what's really missing: *effort*. Like …

– Does he really need to see you in those big, gray pants? Yes, I know they make the line of your clothes look smooth but do both of you a favor and pull them on in privacy.

– Never, ever, EVER let a man see you in pantyhose. I've seen supermodels look dreadful in them and believe me, if they look bad, you're going to look like I do—indescribably terrible.

– This advice has stuck because there is truth in it—you do need to look good for your partner to fancy you. This also means eating well, exercising, and taking pride in your appearance. We all know it's lovely to pull on your sweatpants and snuggle up on the sofa in front of the TV—just get off it occasionally and head to the gym and get dressed up for "dates."

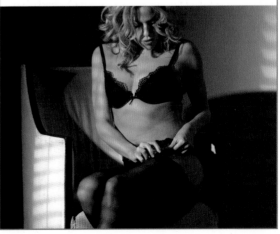

He should be romantic to get more sex

Buy flowers, leave lovey-dovey notes on the fridge, hold her hand, talk to her about her day. That was the standard advice and it probably did work on some, housewifey types who'd hooked up with Neanderthal men, who weren't prone to doing any of this spontaneously. Far more likely to work in reality is—bizarrely ...

- Doing more housework. The more housework a man does, the more sex the couple have— mainly because she's not coming home after working all day to do more work while he puts his feet up in front of the TV.

- Another more effective way to get her to have more sex: make sure it's damn good sex when you do. Try pouncing on her while she's in the shower, for instance. Mix things up a little—not just the location but how you have sex. There's no rule that says you have to touch her breasts first, then use your hands down below, followed by your tongue and then intercourse.

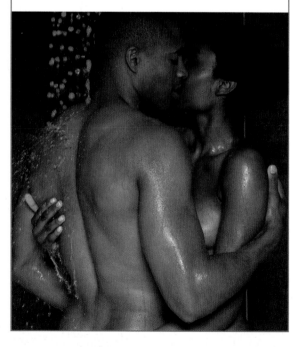

He should have sex like a woman

For years, men have been told to act more like women in bed. Ditch the "wham-bam," guys, and instead spend more time on foreplay, make her feel safe and comfortable, and understand that women are like tiny rosebuds that need gentle coaxing before they open their "petals" and burst into flower. Christ, you were practically told to start every sex session with a full-body aromatherapy massage, pre-ceded by a two-hour chat about "the relationship." Oh, and rose petals scattered on the sheets are mandatory, even on Monday nights. Everybody took this advice on board—and the affair rate climbed higher. That worked then. Not.

The reason why it didn't is that if you ask most people what their best ever sex was, they rarely say, "The time my husband of 10 years ran a bath, gave me a massage, and gently made love to me in bed." Instead it's "Screwing a man I'd just met in the toilet on a plane" or "This gorgeous Swedish girl giving me oral sex in an alley." Hot, urgent, naughty, erotic sex that's usually with someone you shouldn't be with, in a place you shouldn't have sex in, doing something you don't normally do. Danger is what keeps sex red hot long term—this is why couples that are really close friends have problems sustaining desire over time (see pages 106–115).

Clearly, there are some "female" sex traits men do need to pay attention to but there's lots about the male approach to sex that women can learn from. Grabbing it when you can. Not expecting every sex session to last for ages. Having dirty sex and saying "Screw it if the neighbors see or hear." The male sexual psyche might be morally murkier than hers is, but that's not necessarily a bad thing. Women can get too hung up on the whole what's "right" and "wrong" thing! It's not a bad idea to have sex like a gay man either (see pages 126-132).

Men were told to start every sex session with a full-body massage, *pre*-ceded by a two-hour chat about "the relationship."

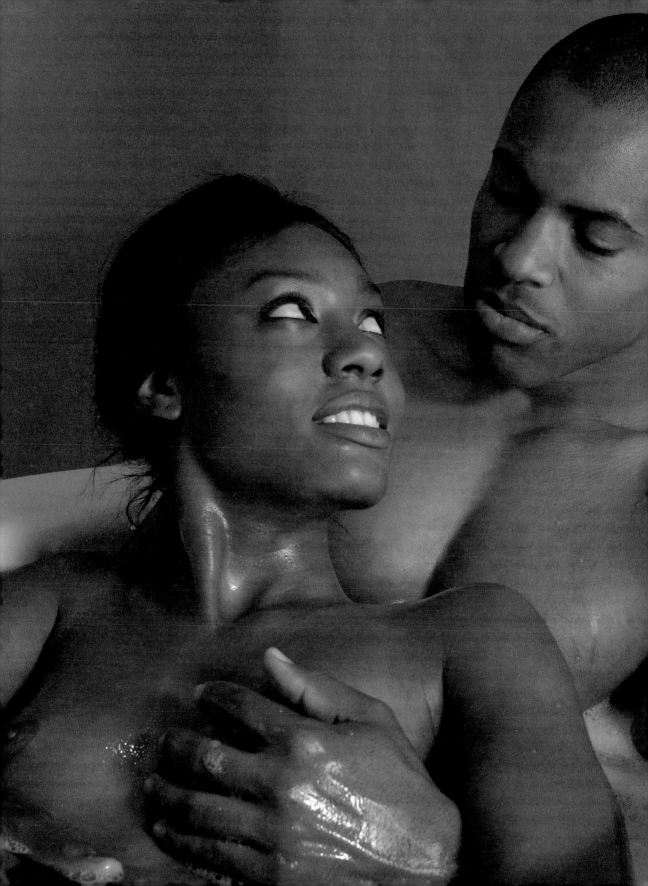

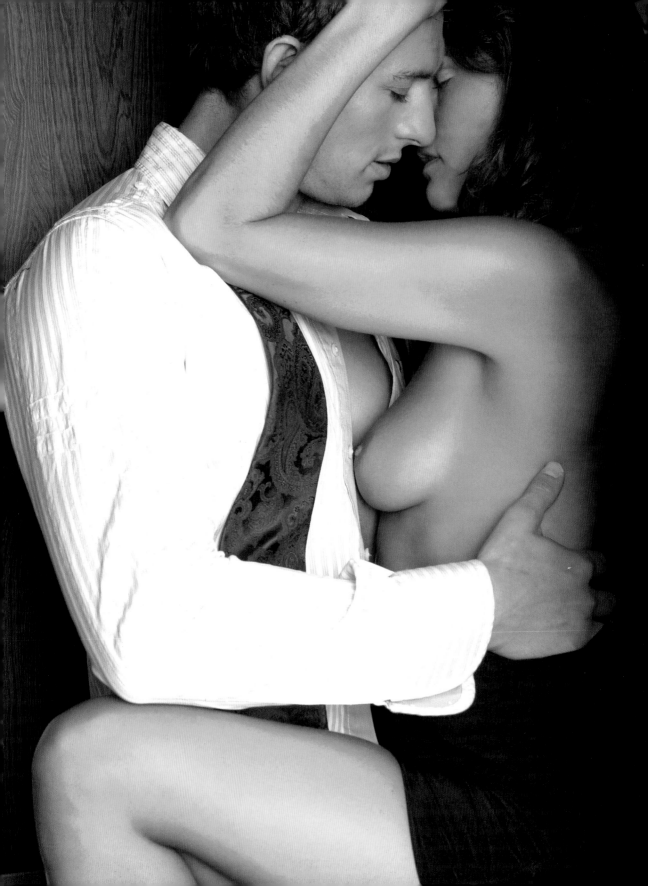

Coming Of Age: Who's Doing What, When

It's easy to tell if you're keeping up with the Joneses with things you can see—not so obvious when sex is something (most) people do behind closed doors. Just how many partners, places, and erotic adventures is normal for a sexually savvy 20-, 30-, and 40-year-old? You're about to find out ...

- Your career's going well, finances under control, and you have both feet firmly planted on the property ladder. But what about your sex life? Would your sexual résumé make your friends jealous with a long list of enviable lovers and wickedly adventurous erotic pursuits? Or would they secretly snigger if they knew what you'd got up to and with whom, smugly patting themselves on the back knowing they'd done *so* much more. Sure, the odd snippets get confessed at drunken dinner parties but it's a brave crowd who'll go into specifics, listing where they've done it, what they've tried, and how many people were there at the time—let alone nitty-gritty specifics about what happened at the lap-dancing club or how they're coping with herpes five years on.

While everybody is different and life choices play a huge part in creating our sexual histories (your list of lovers is going to be far lower if you got married at age 19 rather than 39), there are certain things the average reasonably attractive, sexually liberated, popular person gets up to at a certain age. Some of the conclusions I've drawn here are based on stats from sex research centers like The Kinsey Institute and the infamous Durex Global Sex Survey. Others are based on research from an assortment of various, random sources that I've found to be consistently accurate over the years (believe me, there's a lot of stuff out there that isn't). I've then made some judgement calls based on 15 years of researching, writing, and talking about sex. Because of my job, I know a lot of sexual secrets about a lot of people. None that I would dream of divulging (not even after 10 champagnes—so don't even try) but they do provide real insight into what we all get up to, collectively.

I'm making some presumptions here—that you're attractive, have decent social skills, get to meet a variety of people, are reasonably gregarious, and don't have any major sexual hang-ups. OK, enough justifying. This, boys and girls, is what I think someone like you will probably get up to at a certain point in your life.

In your 20s

- **He can't stop thinking about sex**. Eighty-five percent of 20–30-year-old men think about sex every couple of hours.

- **She's had same-sex fantasies or been bi-curious.** Imagining what it would be like to make love to another woman is nearly always one of the top three female fantasies. Statistically, only 4 percent of women check the "had a lesbian experience" box in surveys but in my experience, it's way, way higher than that. Just as highly educated people are more likely to dip a toe into "kinky" sex, the better educated and more affluent the

20s

Bi-curious experiences, sex-obsessed, adventurous intercourse, no-strings sex, threesomes, sex while high.

30s

Lots of sex alfresco, lots of oral, blindfolds, spanking, tying-up, "Help, the kids stole my sex life," more orgasms.

40s

Less frequent but higher-quality sex, erection problems, infidelity, unsafe sex ... and we're meant to get wiser?

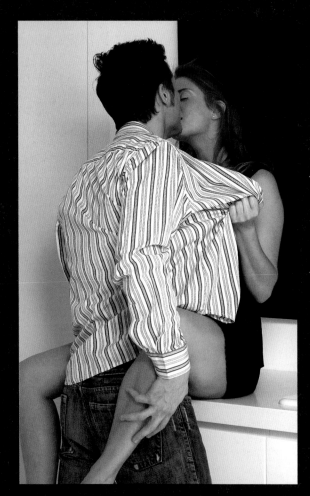

female, the more likely she is to have locked lips with a girl. There's certainly plenty of incentive: a 2006 study of nearly 20,000 people discovered 76 percent of women who slept with women reached orgasm (for women with men, you're pushing to hit 50 percent). Lesbians are also the least promiscuous group and consistently report the highest level of sexual satisfaction. (Remind me why I'm straight again?)

— **Almost everyone's tried "The Wheelbarrow."** This is the age and stage where most of us experiment with positions—the more athletic and unusual, the better! This is also the time when she'll be most likely to attempt to "deep throat" (see page 45).

— **About one in 10 people have had a threesome** in their lifetime. And most of you did it in your early 20s. Threesomes and moresomes aren't quite as common as you think. The majority of people who've had them try them once or twice, then go back to one-on-one sex. The less you know the people involved, the more likely you are to see it as a positive experience. It's also likely you'll visit a strip club or lap-dancing club—with your friends but increasingly often with your partner—at some point in your 20s.

— **About a quarter of you have had sex on drugs.** Senses pleasantly dulled by a puff or glitteringly sharp due to a sniff, about a quarter to maybe a third of you have tried sex while high. Some of you enjoyed it, others didn't. Ecstasy, for instance, is a love drug so plenty get "the cuddles" rather than "the horn," and spend the time rubbing noses and touching foreheads rather than feverishly removing clothes. Coke might put you in the mood—but with a frustratingly unsatisfying end result because he often can't get an erection and it may mean you can't have an orgasm. Smoke a joint and you'll certainly slow up your sex sessions (always a good thing). Sadly, it's sometimes slowed up so much, you both totally forget what you're doing and end up falling asleep in the middle of it (not so good).

In your 30s

Almost all of you have had sex outside. A throwback to our teens—when we all did most of our sexual experimentation behind the garage, in the woods, or in the back of a car—most of us will have sex somewhere semi-public in our 30s. Under the cover of darkness in a park, on a beach, or in your own backyard are top choices. Water sports (but not that kind) are also common. Sex in the shower is pretty much a given and sex in a hot tub is also most likely to happen now, mainly because we've got the money to afford destinations and hotels that have them!

Some form of bondage, blindfolds, and playful spanking has been tried by around 20 percent of you. Either you or your partner have had your hands tied together or to a chair or that hotel four-poster bed (picked exactly for that reason) on a dirty weekend away. Lots will continue to enjoy tying each other up but only five to 10 percent of the population will go on to more serious S&M.

She'll have several gay male friends. Straight women love gay men; gay men love straight women. Why? Well, we're more alike than you think! Swedish research is confirming just why the two groups get along so famously—we both have symmetrical brains. Straight men and lesbians have asymmetrical brain hemispheres. Not only is this more evidence that sexual orientation is not a choice—it may be attributed in part to neurobiology—it explains why nearly all discerning, sage, city-living straight women count at least one or two gay men as their best friends.

One-night stands

Forty-four percent of adults worldwide have had a one-night stand—though it's likely he enjoyed it more than she did.

– A recent poll found that just under half of the women who'd done the walk of shame said it had been a bad idea, four out of five of the men said they'd thoroughly enjoyed their one-time fling with a stranger. Here, in a sentence, is why this might be: he ends up with an orgasm; she ends up with regrets.

– The very essence of having a one-night stand is that it's selfish sex. You're both there for a good time, not a long time, so it's a little unrealistic to expect him to spend two hours trying to give her the pleasure it takes him three minutes to achieve.

– The only way to redress the balance is for her to take control. She should tell him exactly what she wants and how she wants it, satisfying herself first (second, third) before letting him even *think* about his needs.

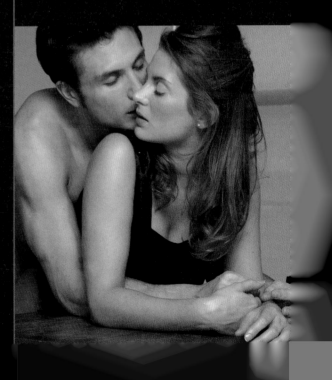

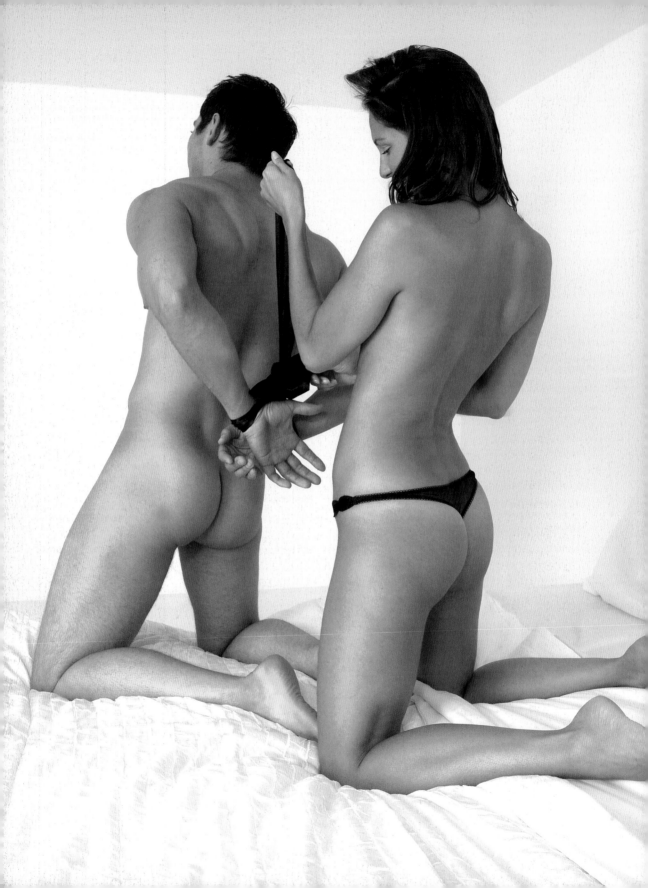

The number of women in their early 30s who've received oral sex is 87 percent. The remaining 13 percent are standing on a cliff ready to jump.

− **You'll have kids—and kiss your sex life goodbye.** Or will you? According to recent research, it's actually not that bad. During pregnancy couples have sex four to five times a month. Most stop for seven weeks after the birth but four months later are back to four to five times a month. Breastfeeding doesn't appear to affect the amount of sex couples have. Six months after the birth, the average couple then have sex three to five times a month. So that's the official stats—but I don't believe them. Judging by the hundreds of letters I receive on the topic and talking to friends and friends of friends, these stats aren't reflecting real life. My personal estimate would be that most couples have sex about once a month while their kids are really young, and sex doesn't really return to normal for about two years. The trick to getting through? Don't pretend it's not happening. Instead, reassure each other it's a temporary glitch, keep touching and cuddling, and when you do have sex, have quickies.

− **Her orgasm quota rises.** Ninety percent of women post 30 regularly experience orgasm, compared to just 23 percent of younger women. Most of them will be achieved via masturbation and oral sex—which is why cunnilingus now features heavily in most sex sessions. One survey found, on average, married women rate oral sex as the most enjoyable way to have an orgasm. Just as anal sex used to be considered terribly "kinky" not so long ago but is now something lots of couples unashamedly enjoy, oral sex was also once considered to be risqué. In the 1930s, only 44 percent of women had ever received oral sex. Today, the number of women in their early 30s who've received oral sex is 87 percent. (The remaining 13 percent are standing on a cliff ready to jump.)

In your 40s

− **More than half of men** will have had problems getting an erection. Up to 52 percent of men between the age of 40 and 70 will find their penises suddenly have a mind of their own. ED (erectile dysfunction) is definitely age related: 39 percent of men aged 40 and above have some form of ED, rising to 67 percent of men aged 70 and over.

− **Almost half of you will have been unfaithful.** The official statistics range between 22 and 41 percent but I'm leaning toward the higher figure as the more accurate. Sorry. Close your eyes for what's to follow because it is depressing. Even people who rated themselves as "pretty happy" with their marriage, cheat. They're twice as likely to have had an affair as those who have "very happy" marriages. Those who report "not too happy" marriages are three times more likely than the "very happy" to have an affair. Only 25 percent of men in another study said they'd had "lots of marital problems" before an affair compared to 48 percent of women. So how happy is happy enough to ward off extramarital temptation? The problem, according to some experts, is that we're pursuing "ultra-happiness," expecting our lives to be ridiculously romantic and sex-fueled, when real life can't possibly measure up. The factors that make us more likely to be unfaithful? You're high risk if you've been together a long time, have had a high number of partners prior to your relationship, you're male, live in a city, and/or think about sex several times a day.

− **You're most likely to have unsafe sex.** Research proves people 40 plus are the worst at observing even the basics of safe sex! STIs have doubled in under a decade in people over 45 and are now rising faster than with teenagers. Assuming only young people have sexually transmitted infections is about as stupid as thinking "nice" people couldn't possibly have any. Then there's pregnancy. You might decide you're finished having children post 40, but unless you use contraception, your body might have other ideas. The same rules apply for you as your teenage kids: use a condom every single time you have sex and if you're in a monogamous relationship, both get tested for STIs at a sexual health clinic before ditching the condoms completely. Be aware the only true safe sex is

The mile-high club

Despite the hype that surrounds the mile-high club, only 2 percent of adults have actually plucked up the nerve to do it.

- Be warned, it is illegal. Be discreet about it and don't leave any signs of what you've been up to. Choose a night flight, where the cabin lights are dimmed and most passengers are asleep.

- Having decided on a signal of when to open the door, one of you disappears to the toilet. The other waits a few minutes, then goes to stand by the door. Wait for your moment, then knock, and then walk inside as usual.

- While there, time is limited. One of you gets oral sex, or she leans forward over the seat, he enters from behind. You won't know if you've got away with it until you come out. If there's someone waiting while the first person exits, you're busted—in which case, apologize, flash a cheeky grin, and hope they've got a sense of humor. The person who walks out second will be the most humiliated, but if it was fun, who cares?

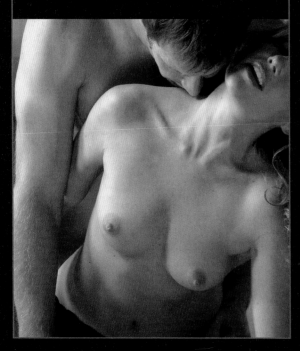

abstinence—condoms don't protect you against everything and there's no guarantee a partner will be faithful. It's all a bit of a judgement call—so just make sure it's a good one.

- **You're having sex less than ever before**—but the good news is it's better quality. Eighteen to 29-year-olds have sex an average of 112 times a year, 30–39 year olds around 86 times a year. Blow out that last candle on your 40th birthday cake and (if you haven't passed out from the effort) your average drops to 69. No need to be too depressed though: the frequency decreases but satisfaction levels rise.

- **Nearly a third of all married men will be regularly watching porn on the net.** Men make up two-thirds of the users of sexually explicit internet sites and account for 77 percent of online time. Most women will have checked out internet porn by their 40s. Despite the high level of interest, few people (just 1 percent) become addicted. Of those that are, though, 38 percent are married men. I have to say every man I know over the age of 16 admits to checking out internet porn regularly. You can pretend all you like that it's a fad that's going to go away but it *soooooooo* isn't. For more on Net Sex, see pages 132–135.

So what happens when we get older? The really good news is that sex gets better. Recent research compared modern day with a 1971 survey and found those over 70 are enjoying more sex than ever before! Sixty-eight percent of married men said they're still enjoying sex, compared to just 52 percent back then. Fifty-six percent of married women also said they were also happy with their sex lives compared to the previous 38 percent.

Lesbians are also the least promiscuous group and consistently report the highest level of sexual satisfaction. (Remind me why I'm straight again?)

The official sex stats

How often?
Men have sex 104 times per year, women have it 101. One in five adults has sex 3–4 times a week and 5 percent have sex once a day. Reports vary on figures for each age group but there's actually not that much difference in frequency from when you're aged 20 to when you hit 45—they all hover between 108 and 112.

Horniest nation?
The Greeks appear to have sex the most at 138 times per year, the Japanese have it the least at 45 times a year. (This is blamed on exhaustion from commuting, high work stress, long working hours, and small living spaces that couples often share with parents.)

Who's obsessed with it?
Fifty-four percent of men think about sex every day or several times a day compared to 19 percent of women.

When do we lose it?
The average age of first intercourse is at 16.9 for men and at 17.4 for women.

Who's straight, gay, and bi?
Ninety percent of 18–44-year-old men consider themselves straight, 2.3 percent gay, 1.8 percent bi, and 3.8 percent as "something else" (hello?). Ninety percent of 18–44-year-old women also consider themselves straight with 1.3 percent gay, 2.8 percent bi, and 3.8 percent "something else." Twenty percent of gay men have been heterosexually married.

When are we most likely to marry?
We tend to marry for the first time in our late 20s or very early 30s. Once we tie the knot, 45 percent have sex a few times per month. Thirty-four percent have it two to three times a week and only seven percent four or more times a week. Thirteen percent of married men and 12 percent of married women had only had sex a few times in the past year.

How many partners?
Globally, condom-maker Durex says the average for men and women is nine in a lifetime (10.2 for men and 6.9 for women). This has risen from the 2005 Kinsey research that came up with four partners for women and six to eight for men.

Rate of masturbation?
Ninety-eight percent of men and 44 percent of women have masturbated. Men DIY a dozen times per month, women around five times. Nearly 85 percent of men and 45 percent of women who live with a sexual partner still masturbate solo.

Where are we doing it?
Outside bed, the most common place is the car (50 percent), followed by the bathroom (39 percent), our parents' bedroom (36 percent), and a park (31 percent). Only 15 percent of people have had sex at work. Twenty-two percent of Americans and Canadians have had sex in front of a camera.

Are we happy with our sex lives?
Forty-four percent of adults are happy with their sex life. Men are the least satisfied with how often they have sex— 41 percent want it more frequently, compared to 29 percent of women. Four in 10 want new ideas about sex.

What pleases women?
Women are more likely to orgasm solo than with a partner. Seventy-five percent of men and 29 percent of women always have orgasms with their partner.

Who has the safest sex?
Women are slightly less likely to take risks than men— 45 percent to his 48 percent. The older you are, the more likely you are to have unprotected sex— by a substantial percentage. Greeks, Norwegians, and Swedes are the least likely to wear a condom; people from India, Hong Kong, and Spain the most likely.

Sex On The Brain

Think you're in charge of your love and sex life? Think again. When we call people "love junkies," we are actually being accurate: we're all completely and utterly under the influence of our brain hormones.

Whether it's just a lustful look, a one-night stand, or marriage and babies—we like to kid ourselves it's our decision what form and path our relationships take. Think again. In fact, we might as well relinquish all responsibility, throw our hands and panties in the air, and leave our love lives in the lap of the Gods. You think *you're* choosing who you fall in love with? Who you fall *out* of love with? When, where, and how? Hah! It's brain hormones not your head, heart, or other parts deciding your future. Logic and sensibility don't stand a chance against the army of sex and love chemicals, hormones, and neurotransmitters released during attraction, lust, and love by our brain. And they're as volatile and argumentative as they are potent, each jostling with the other for control. Is it any wonder the path of true love doesn't run smoothly with this lot at the controls?

The chemicals that are released during infatuation are the same ones triggered when someone cheats and a drug addict gets their fix. To say they're powerful stuff is such an understatement; it's a bit like saying letting off a nuclear bomb might do a little bit of damage. "The brain is a chemical factory looking for love," says Daniel Amen, world-prominent neuroscientist. Anthropologist Helen Fisher warns, "Do not copulate with people you do not want to fall in love with, because you might do just that." If you're not quaking in your boots, you should be. We are "love junkies"—completely under the influence of brain hormones. Sex bonds you to others but then even a simple glance at a pretty or handsome stranger can instigate a chemical reaction that's instant and bogglingly mind-altering. If you want half a chance of going the distance as a couple, you need to arm yourself with these neurological facts. At the very least, knowing what the three phases of love and sex are means you can anticipate what you're in for.

Attraction

You see, you want. And what you want is usually young, healthy, and symmetrical. Men are programmed to look for fertile women (small waist, curvy hips); women are programmed to seek good providers (big wallet, sports car). Fifty percent of our brain is dedicated to vision, which is why looks are so important initially.

The chemical cocktail

- **Testosterone** is mainly produced by his testicles but her ovaries also create a small amount. It's responsible for sex drive. Estrogen is produced primarily in her ovaries but both his and her brain also manufacture it. It regulates the menstrual cycle but also helps to maintain a healthy, lubricated vagina.

- **Nitric oxide** is released by our genitals when we're aroused. This is what causes blood vessels to dilate, allowing more blood to pump to crucial parts—like his penis. Impotency drugs Viagra and Cialis (see pages 33–34) work by stimulating the release of nitric oxide.

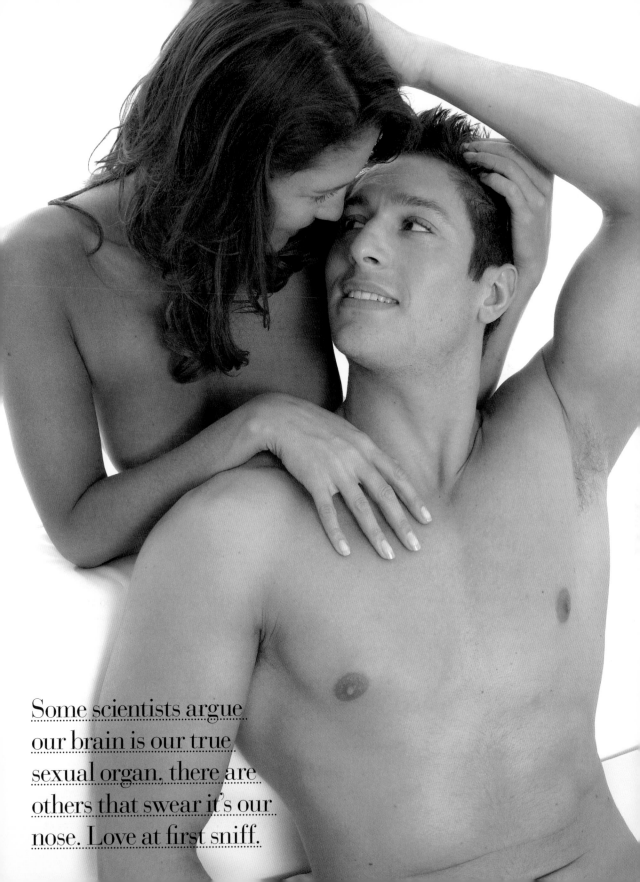

Some scientists argue
our brain is our true
sexual organ. there are
others that swear it's our
nose. Love at first sniff.

– **Pheromones** are scented hormones that are secreted by our sweat glands, chiefly under our arms, and researchers are still pondering exactly how they work. What is clear is that they're crucial in deciding who we want to get horizontal with and who we don't. The scent they emit is vital: numerous experiments have shown if someone doesn't smell good to us, we won't go there. In fact, as much as some scientists argue our brain is our true sexual organ, there are others that swear it's our nose. Love at first sniff.

Potential problems
None if you're both single and attracted to each other. Huge if one or both of you are involved with someone else. This mix of chemicals and hormones is potent with a capital P. Caught in the grips of it, like a rabbit caught in headlights, thoughts of the long-term consequences caused by acting on desire are obliterated. Look away, move away, hit yourself over the head with a heavy object—just do whatever it takes to break the spell.

Infatuation

You got what you wanted and have embarked on some kind of relationship. This is the "honeymoon" period, the "in love", dippy, swooning bit. The part when you can't think of anything but the person you've just met. If they dropped on one knee and asked you to elope in the first two weeks, you'd say yes. You're either manically happy when they show your feelings are reciprocated or in total, abject despair if they call five minutes later than they promised to. The word "obsessive" hardly begins to describe how often they pop into your head.

The chemical cocktail
– **Epinephrine and norepinephrine –** neurotransmitters produced in the adrenal glands, spinal cord, and brain. They're called "excitatory neurotransmitters" because that's exactly what they do: create tummy flip-flops, a fast beating heart, and an adrenaline rush of excitement. This keeps us aroused and also helps push us over the edge into orgasm.

– **Dopamine** is the undisputed star of the neuro-transmitters associated with infatuation because it controls the big three: pleasure, motivation, and concentration. It's the boss of the "reward center"

of our brain, giving us a kick up the bottom to seek out pleasure and making sure we enjoy it when we do by focusing on the task at hand.

– **Serotonin**, the "feel good" neurotransmitter produced in the mid-brain, controls our mood and emotions and how flexible we are in our thinking. Bizarrely, considering it's nicknamed the "happy chemical," we'll often have low levels of it when first in love. This is why we often feel moody and anxious as well as ecstatic.

– **PEA (phenylethylamine)** acts a bit like adrenaline by speeding up the flow of information between nerve cells. PEA ensures we pay attention to all the "love" feelings and gives the nod for chemicals to flood into the brain, creating feelings of euphoria.

Potential problems
Dopamine and serotonin battle during infatuation because the higher the level of dopamine, the lower the level of serotonin. They can't coexist at the same level. This means in one corner, we have dopamine trying desperately to make us behave in a way that's lovable; in the other corner, low serotonin—forcing us to make bad judgement calls because of obsessive thinking – does its best to make us unlikeable. PEA can play havoc if you're already attached and someone other than your partner has you quivering with pleasure. It makes us impulsive—and prone to shag first, think (about losing the wife/husband/kids/house) later. Too late type of later.

Commitment

If you've managed to survive the emotional rollercoaster that is infatuation, you'll move into the "true love" stage. It's calmer and less crazed than the other two but this doesn't mean it's any less intense. This is when you feel a sense of connection, a quiet happiness, and feel at peace with the world. It's also the time when sexual desire also puts its feet up and kicks back. Who can be bothered having sex when you're quite content snuggling on the sofa watching TV with some take-out?

The chemical cocktail
– **Oxytocin** is released by the pituitary gland and acts on the ovaries and testes to regulate reproduction. More importantly, it's the bonding, "cuddle" chemical. When

you hold hands or hug the person you love, oxytocin levels soar along with your heart. Our levels shoot up during sex, peaking at orgasm, but his catapult to a level more than 500 percent the usual after he's had one! Considering this is also the hormone that is released during breastfeeding, designed to make babies sleep afterward, it could explain why men want to nod off when women have just got going. Oxytocin also has an amnesiac effect during sex and orgasm in that it blocks negative memories people have about each other. Yet another reason why couples that have lots of sex actually like each other more. High oxytocin levels are also associated with trust. What's not to like about this one?

– **Vasopressin** is found in higher levels in his brain than hers—which isn't surprising since it's in charge of "male" behaviors like dominance, sexual persistence, and territorial feelings. It's also lovey-dovey and releases when he's in *lurve*.

Potential problems

Again, it's the differing hormone levels that can create havoc. Once there are high levels of oxytocin and vasopressin, dopamine and norepinephrine pathways are compromised. So infatuation bids a sad farewell as attachment increases. The relationship feels less exciting because of it. Even worse, while elevated levels of vasopressin in men makes him feel all fuzzy, protective, and loving, the downside is it affects his sex drive. The more in love he is, the more vasopressin there is in his system, which causes levels of testosterone (which make him feel like sex) to reduce. In plain English, the more attached he feels, the less likely he is to want to screw you senseless. Brilliant.

PEA can create havoc. It makes us impulsive—and prone to shag first, think (about losing the wife/ husband/kids/house) later. Too late type of later.

Trick your brain

Here's how to get the better of those hormones ...

– Forget everything you've been told. "Trust, familiarity, predictability, romance—are not the building blocks of desire, says sex therapist Ian Kerner.

– Be a thrillseeker. Novelty is what tricks the brain into producing the hormones it did at the start. Push yourselves out of your comfort zones, rather than stay where you feel safe. Feed your fantasies. Be naughty. Think edgy.

– Don't live in each other's pockets. If you have sex with and see your partner all the time, there's no need for dopamine because you don't have to work hard to get a reward. Being separated makes our brain sit up and pay attention.

– There's an argument for arguing. Make-up sex is hot because anger stimulates the production of adrenaline, which in turn produces dopamine. A huge row also puts the relationship at risk, making us appreciate the person we almost lost.

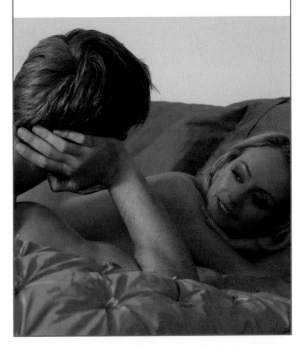

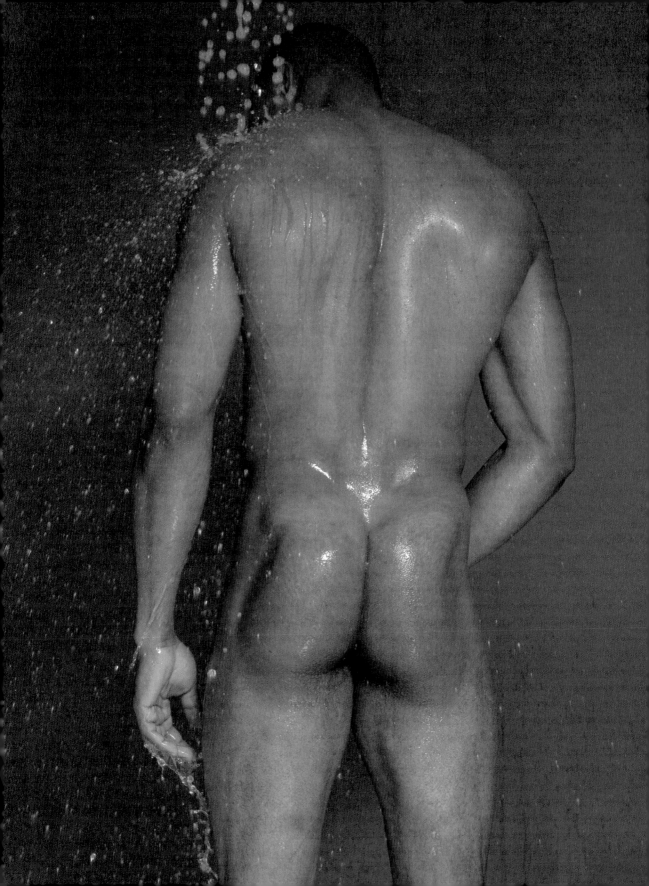

Stiff Competition

It's an object of worship, yet causes more anxiety than any other body part. Myths about the male member abound, so let's dispel a few, shall we? This one's for the boys—but girls will get BIG brownie points by boning up on his favorite topic.

Answer me honestly: if there was one question you could ask all your girlfriends, past and present, what would it be? I'd wager a bet it's this one: "How big/wide/hard is my penis, compared to other guys?" (followed closely by, "And how am I in bed?"). Just how much men base their sexual self-esteem on their penis never fails to astound me. (Though, you're not the only one who thinks it's your most important part: the tissue that surrounds the penis is more durable than the tissue that surrounds the brain!) I have to say, I get it. I get the pride and I get the paranoia. And, as I'm very fond of saying, I'm very glad I don't own one.

Penises sometimes have a mind of their own— and, diabolically, every decision it makes is visible. Women can fake almost everything (lube for arousal, a few moans for orgasm), but what's happening with you is far more obvious. Which is why you need to let go of that ridiculous assumption that a) you can control your penis (you can't), and b) that it should behave like it does in the (porn) movies. Give the poor little (sorry, big) fella a chance. He's not a robot, he's human. And just like you, he gets tired, stressed, overexcited, and/or distinctly underwhelmed by things.

You may have had unpleasant experiences with women reacting badly when your penis hasn't behaved exactly as it "should." But often that's because you freak out and she takes her cue from you. Or she's fallen for the same "perfect penis" myth because men try to hide it from women when things aren't going so well.

The more honest you are with your partner about the quirky ups and downs that come with owning a penis, the less concerned she's going to be if things don't go to plan sometimes. Besides, in 99—no, let's make that 100—percent of cases the reason she's alarmed is because she thinks it's her fault. She's too fat/her breasts aren't big enough/you don't fancy her, blah blah blah. (Something else to remember: if she likes you, she'll definitely like your penis.)

All easily solved by you taking a vow—one hand on your penis, the other on your heart—that, from now on, you will swear to tell the truth, the whole truth and nothing but the truth about your penis and how it behaves to your partner and any future partners. That's a huge step in the right direction. As for the rest of the wobbles, hopefully the following will help ...

Guys, remember, there is such a thing as a "good enough" erection. They don't all have to resemble Rambo's forearm

How it all works

The penis is a fleshy appendage that, when limp, curls against the lower abdomen. Excited, it springs to attention and lengthens and thickens until it sticks out at an upward angle from the belly.

- Despite it feeling rock hard (well, it does if you're 18), there aren't any bones in the penis—the rigidity is caused simply by blood pumping ferociously into the three cylinders inside it.

- There are two larger, pencil-like cylinders on the top (looking from above) and one underneath. The urethra, the tube through which urine and sperm pass, runs through the bottom cylinder. The cylinders are held together by what's been nicknamed "industrial strength cling wrap" (Buck's fascia). The upper cylinders are spongy and have their own artery, allowing the sponges to fill up with blood, which gives you an erection.

- Veins are clearly visible across the upper surface and the "main switchboard" of the nerve supply is also here, but because it breaks off into mini networks, the whole organ experiences pleasure.

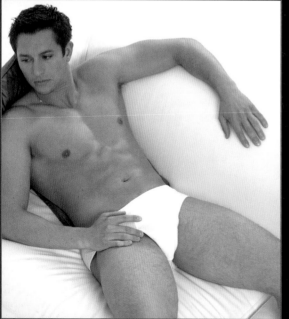

The erection section

Types of erection

- **The first type** of erection comes courtesy of the brain: it's called a psychogenic erection and it's produced when the brain recognizes erotic stimuli—both real or imagined. If you're bored with sex, this is the erection that will be most affected.

- **The second type** is a reflex erection, which results from direct genital stimulation. Stress and depression can interfere with this guy.

- **The third type** is a nocturnal erection, the least effort variety that you get spontaneously during REM (rapid eye movement) sleep. This erection is significant. If you're not getting the other two but are waking up "pee proud," the cause is probably psychological rather than physical. Most men get around seven erections a day—five of them are nocturnal.

Rate your erection

If they were asked to rate their erection, most guys would probably only have two ratings—up and down. Sex therapists are a little more specific, rating them on a scale of 1–10. It's useful in a diagnostic sense but also helps clients move from the "all or nothing/success or failure" model to a sensible, "I have a 6 today. Excellent!" way of thinking. There is such a thing as a "good enough" erection, they don't all have to resemble Rambo's forearm. Try thinking like this: If 0 is no erection at all, you're a 1 when blood starts to trickle in, climbing to a 2, 3, 4, or 5 when enough blood's in there.

It then gets progressively harder turning it into a 6, 7 and working it's way through to 10. Your *personal* version of the hardest erection is a 10—we're not comparing it to Long Dong Silver's 10. (Or are we? The infamous porn star reputedly had a 18-inch /45-cm penis that took so much blood to fill, it never did get fully erect. We now know the actor used to wear a prosthetic penis, but it's still a great story!) Most erections move up the scale during a normal sex session. The more direct stimulation the penis gets, the harder it remains. It's OK if you need physical stimulation to get an erection. Some guys get one by looking at something sexy, others need to be touched. It's also possible to be aroused, but not have an erection. You can actually orgasm without an erection!

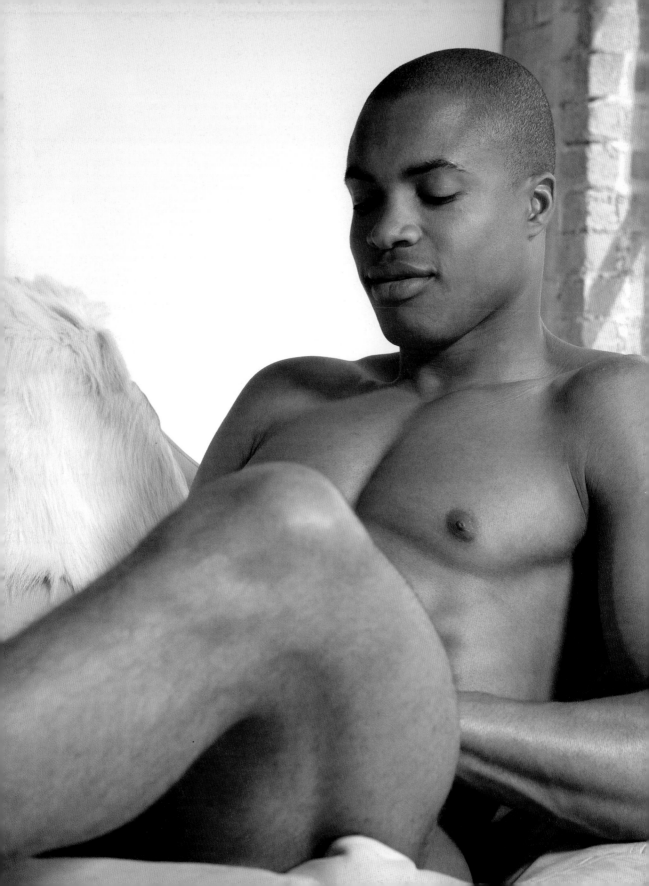

1

Trim your pubic hair—your penis will look bigger, and she'll be more inclined to give you oral. Losing that tummy will also make your penis look bigger.

2

To make sure you last that bit longer, pop on a condom to reduce sensation or masturbate just before the session starts.

3

If you lose your erection with condoms, try wearing larger and thinner ones, plus add a penis ring or vibrating penis ring to hold it all in place.

4

Think twice before lighting that ciggie. Smokers are twice as likely as non-smokers to suffer from impotency.

Dinner party dazzlers

Forget chatting about the weather, politics, or your job. Slip some penis trivia into the conversation and watch the party stand up and pay attention …

– Teenage erections last up to an hour. The average guy aged 20–40 can keep an erection for around 40 minutes. Aged 66–70, you're lucky to last seven.

– If you've got large testicles, you're more likely to cheat and will want sex 30 percent more than other "average" guys. Well, that's what one study found.

– Two in every thousand men can give themselves fellatio. The quality, however, is debatable given the contorted position needed to achieve this.

– The more often you have sex, the less likely you'll be to have erection problems. Having lots of sex keeps your penis healthy. Erections flood the penis with oxygen-rich blood and oxygen keeps the muscle tissue inside healthy. A shortage of oxygen can lead to a build-up of collagen, which in turn affects your erection. One study of 1,000 men aged 55–75 in Finland found that men who had sex less than once a week were twice as likely to develop erectile dysfunction as men who had sex at least once a week.

– Between half and one teaspoon of semen is what the average man ejaculates. If you're super-healthy and super-hydrated, you'll do this in 3–10 spurts, about 0.8 seconds apart at a speed of around 25–28 miles an hour. Aged 15–60, the average man will ejaculate 30–50 quarts (28–47 liters) of semen containing 350–500 billion sperm cells.

– Circumcision does not reduce the risks of penile cancer or STIs. That old chestnut was fed to parents who questioned the sensibility of cutting off their sons' foreskins. The practice continues in the US. There is one beneficiary of circumcision—science. Hundreds of thousands of discarded foreskins have been sold to pharmaceutical companies and research labs for clinical research.

Penis problems

What happens if I lose my erection during sex?

The same myth that says you will always get an erection on cue and ejaculate the second you want to also says men get an erection at the start of a sex session and maintain it at that level of hardness all the way through. Never mind if you've spent 20 intense, unselfish minutes giving her oral, never mind her going off to the bathroom for a quick pee, never mind your cell-phone text alert going off, you're supposed to stay rock hard throughout. Aren't you? What do *you* think?

Listen, it's normal to get harder, softer, really hard, even harder, sort of medium soft, almost lose it, then get really hard before you orgasm. The amount of blood in the penis affects how hard you are and it's driven by arousal. You don't stay at *exactly* the same level of excitement during a sex session, so it's logical your penis won't either. Most of the time, you won't even notice this happening but if you do notice your erection going down, don't panic. Your natural inclination will be to tense up. Don't—it cuts off the blood flow, which is what causes your erection. Instead, relax into it. Focus. Relax your penis and the muscles around it. Take a break and pleasure her to take the pressure off and calm down. Then start again, focusing on the sensations you're feeling rather than how hard you are.

What can I do with a semi-erect penis?

You don't have to be hard to have intercourse, even if the "putting it in" part is now referred to as (a rather undignified) "stuffing." Use lube and get in a side-by-side position, like "scissors" (one leg on top, other leg between). Get her to push your penis inside her by pushing the base first—the head naturally follows. Once you're inside, resist the urge to pump furiously, simply stay inside, get her to clench and release her vaginal muscles and do the same with your PC muscles. Simply focus on how nice it feels, kiss, *relax*. Then start to thrust gently and experimentally.

Should I pop a Viagra if I'm worried?

If you have real impotency problems and have been prescribed Viagra by a doctor, sure. Otherwise, I wouldn't recommend it. I know some of you will pop one just to see what happens. And you might end up with a whopping great, wondrously hard erection and have a

Bent as a banana

You won't go blind from excessive masturbation but you might bend your penis. Peyronie's Disease, a bend or curve in the penis, affects up to four percent of the population, commonly men aged 40–60. There is no cure for it at present, but there is ongoing medical research into the condition.

– They don't really know what causes it but it appears to be hereditary or caused by "trauma," which can include "excessive" masturbation or intercourse. If you have it (and you won't know until you see symptoms), it may kick in later in life if you don't keep your penis healthy (see box, opposite). This is why it's important to have regular sex and keep the blood flowing through.

– However, it's not all bad news if you do develop it. A really good friend of mine who is having very good sex with a man who has Peyronie's can testify, it can have benefits. That kink can mean his penis tucks under the pubic bone, perfectly positioned for a direct hit to the G-spot! The bend is also handy for reaching the front wall of the vagina where it wouldn't usually.

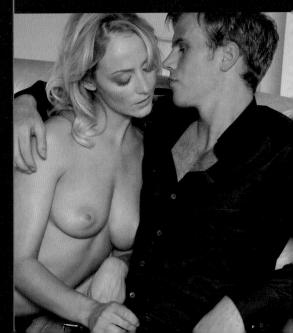

Never mind if you've spent 20 intense, unselfish minutes giving her oral, never mind her going off to the bathroom for a quick pee, you're supposed to stay rock hard throughout.

fabulous time. Or you might just end up with a whopping headache. And if you have heart problems you didn't know about, you might end up in the ER. So it's not worth the risk. (The only safe way to try Viagra is to ask your doctor for some, rather than trawl the internet, because you need a physical before taking them.)

Let's have a little Viagra lesson while we're on the topic. Viagra—nicknamed "potency in a pill"—is the same drug that was used to treat heart disease. It works by inhibiting production of an enzyme, allowing the smooth muscle cells in the penis to relax, making it easier for it to engorge with blood and maintain an erection. You take one an hour before you want some action and it lasts about four hours.

The greatest myth is that taking Viagra will suddenly result in an instant erection. It won't. Take one and do the crossword and absolutely nothing will happen. It only works with stimulation. Viagra also has competitors— Levitra and Cialis. Levitra has fewer side effects (Viagra can cause nausea, indigestion, and headaches) and works quicker. Cialis lasts up to 36 hours, which takes the pressure off having to "do it" within a certain period of time. All very useful to know for when you're past 50, which is when you're most likely to use them.

Can you break a penis?!
No, because there aren't any bones in it but you can do serious damage. I "broke" my ex's penis once. He was aiming for me and instead got the end of the bed— hard wood. Like *owww*. Really *owwww*. He was (miraculously) fine for a few weeks but then one day (the day after Christmas, to be precise) he discovered he couldn't pee. Not ideal when you've just had 50 million Christmas beers, your stomach is swelling, and a purple vein has just popped out the head of your penis.

We hot-footed it to the emergency room and they put in a catheter—turned out the accident had badly kinked his urethra. (He neglected to tell me he'd be peeing in five different directions at once since then.) He's OK, by the way, but accidents can and do happen—usually in this scenario, when an erect penis is thrust against a very hard object. Often you'll hear a crack and your erection will disappear faster than you can say "Help me God!" It might also bend to one side. If this does happen (and I

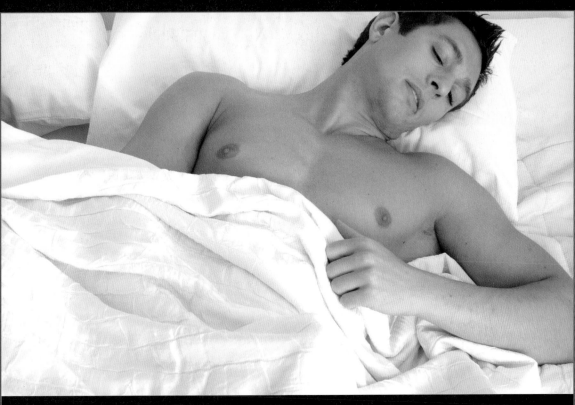

You want quicker or stronger erections?

Dr. Barbara Keesling is a Canadian sex therapist with literal hands-on experience—she worked as a sex surrogate—jumping into bed with couples to fix their sexual problems (and no I haven't and am not likely to anytime soon). Not only is she gorgeous, she gives good sex advice. I can't top her following tips, so these are based on advice in her book *Sexual Pleasure*.

For quicker erections

- There's evidence that slowly massaging the base of the penis and squeezing the shaft, with lube or in the shower for five minutes a day, works. Use the opposite hand that you usually use and you'll be less likely to get aroused. You're massaging not masturbating.

- The idea is to relax your PC muscles: the more relaxed they are, the more your penis will fill with blood. You should see results in about three weeks and notice it takes less time to get aroused.

For stronger erections

- Most men tighten their PC muscle when they feel an erection about to happen. This works momentarily but after that, it does the opposite and constricts the blood flow. The next time you feel your penis start to fill with blood, consciously relax.

- Get your partner to help retrain your penis: she lies on the bed next to you and stimulates you.

- If you feel yourself tense when you start to become erect, tell your partner and get her to stop the stimulation. (Yes, you must, however enjoyable it is!) Consciously relax your PC muscle then get her to continue. Repeat this sequence for a while, then try the technique again the next time.

- Now try doing the same exercise with your penis inside her. Again, stop thrusting and wait for a few seconds before recommencing, consciously relaxing your penis during this time. Get into the habit of doing this even when you're happy with the strength of your erections—it adds tension for both of you.

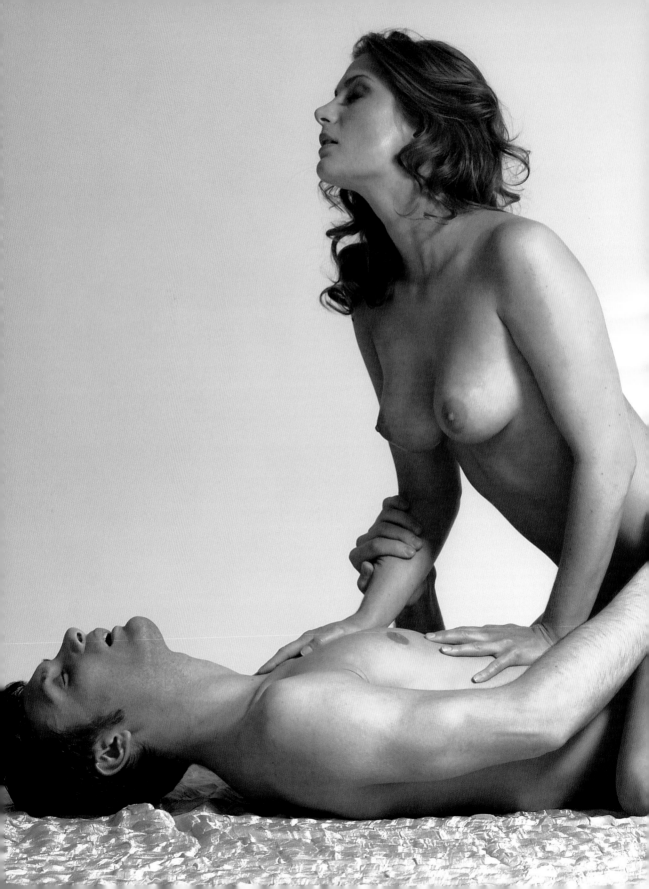

Chapter Two

Doing It

Melt In The Mouth

Oral sex is up there with life's greatest pleasures. The secret to making it really good is simple—you have to enjoy both the giving and receiving.

If you've read any of my other books, you'll know that I'm a bit of an oral sex junkie. OK, maybe more than a bit ... I might have been known to push old ladies out of the way to get to a guy who happens to innocently lick his fingers. But by God, it's nice, isn't it? So nice, you'd sort of sell your soul for it if push came to shove. Which is why it's absolutely crucial you get it right. Giving great oral is part attitude, part technique, and a whole lot about enthusiasm. You'll find how-to guides for both of you here but there are basics that apply to both:

– **It's a treat not a chore.** Treat oral sex like it's a huge favor and the experience will be awful, no matter how practiced your tongue techniques. Giving your partner pleasure should be almost as fulfilling for you as for them. The best oral sessions are offered enthusiastically, not asked for and delivered begrudgingly.

– **Ignore what they do in porn films.** It's totally misleading. In porn movies, they pull back when he's giving her oral so you can see what's going on. In real life you can't normally see what's happening because his face is pressed against you, and it *feels* better like that. And in porn movies girls deep-throat everyone— you don't have to in real life, and guys suck hard on clitorises, pulling them out like they're made of chewing gum. Do *that* in real life and you'll never see her genitals up close and personal again (or her, for that matter).

– **Make sure your bits are lickable.** Shower regularly, keep your pubic hair under control (and, guys, can you please shave before going down on us? Stubble's sexy to look at, not so sexy when it's scraping a layer of skin off our thighs). You could shave or wax off your pubic hair—some people love the look and it makes everything neat, clean, and her clitoris easier to find. Others find it a total turn-off because of the whole "Ew, you look like an adolescent" thing. Do what makes you happy and see what your partner has to say about it.

– **Give each other guidance.** I think a good "let's learn about each other" session works well about the fifth or sixth time you've slept together because you've got over that initial shyness. Start by talking about what you like, then demonstrate. He can suck her finger to show what he likes, she can lick his palm to do the same. Then try it out on your actual bits. Do it with the lights on or in daylight—he, especially, needs to see what he's doing. Instruct, don't order, and be tactful. "That feels great," or "I liked the other way better," works better than, "Stop now. I hate it."

– **It's about connection.** Everyone is individual and to be the best your partner ever had, you've got to be constantly on the alert for their reaction to whatever you're trying. It's good to use different techniques but the main aim is to give that particular person pleasure. Timing is crucial as well.

– **It's got to be reciprocal.** I'm not saying you both have to do each other in the same session but I am saying it should even up over time. If your partner wants you to do it to them but won't ever reciprocate, refuse. It's selfish, unfair, and totally unacceptable.

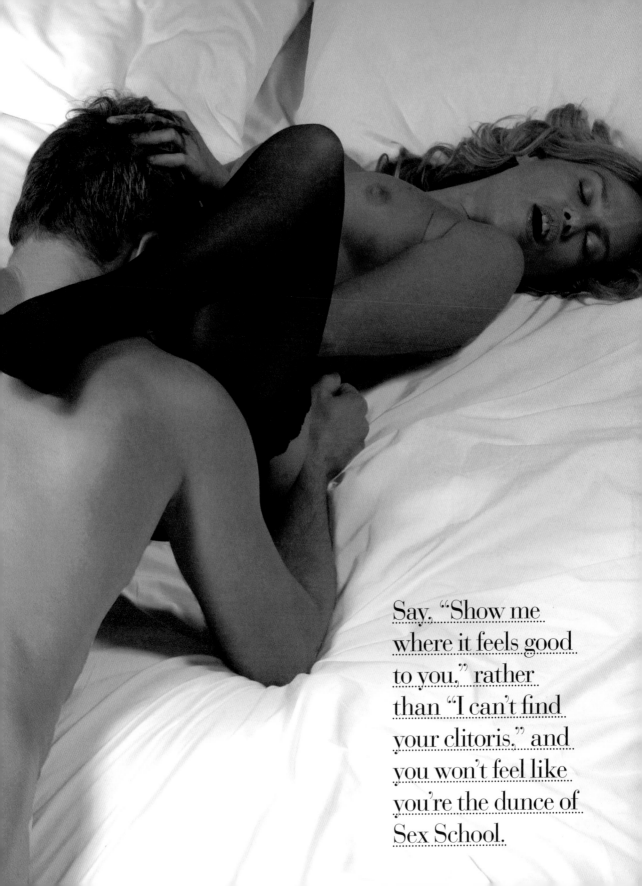

Say, "Show me
where it feels good
to you," rather
than "I can't find
your clitoris," and
you won't feel like
you're the dunce of
Sex School.

Giving her oral

Pick your position

– **She takes ages.** Try her seated, slouched forward in a chair, or sitting on the kitchen worktop. Get her to slide forward, so her crotch is on the edge of the chair or surface. Put pillows under your knees for comfort and to get the height right. This makes it easier on your neck, means you can use your fingers, and see exactly what you're doing. Get her to put her feet on your shoulders or something else close by (though preferably not the dinner you've just cooked).

– **She's fussy or you're unsure what she really wants.** Get her to straddle your face. You're lying on your back, she then climbs on board, facing in either direction (depending on whether you're a breast or bottom man!) and balances by putting her hands on the wall or bedhead. She's got control over everything in this position because she can lift or lower to position herself just so. There's something fabulously filthy about it as well. Put a pillow under your neck and it's quite relaxed, though some guys feel a bit suffocated in this position. If she crouches too low, it can be the female equivalent of you pushing the back of her head.

– **She's self-conscious.** Stick to the traditional pose of her lying on her back, while you lie between her legs. It's relaxing for her, she doesn't feel exposed, and she can do whatever it takes to get there—concentrate/fantasize/recite the alphabet. To make things comfy, put a pillow under her ass and one under your chest.

– **She's begging for it.** She stands, you kneel in front of her. This is perfect for urgent sex plus it appeals to alpha females who like seeing you shamelessly submissive in front of them. If she goes weak at the knees, literally, and can't stand any longer—or can't orgasm standing up (some can't)—get her to lean against a wall or pull her to the floor to continue. Another good position for confident girls: get her on all fours on the bed, then simply slide in underneath, putting your head on pillows so you can reach.

– **You want to impress.** Lie on your back on the bed with your head hanging over the edge and get her to straddle your mouth. Or start in the traditional pose of you between her legs, then get up on your knees and lift her legs so her ankles are on your shoulders, before continuing the job. Another hot favorite: bend her over the sofa, face down, and get her to spread her legs then lick from behind. You need a tongue like a lizard to get there but if you shift around enough, it's do-able.

Take her to heaven

– **Don't just rip her panties off** and bury your face. Instead, lick through her panties. Long, wet, teasing licks. Then push them to one side, get really close—and simply breathe on her for a second or two, followed by one single, deliciously debilitating lick. Tease further by pushing them back into place and continuing to lick through the fabric.

– **Peel her knickers off** totally and take a moment to just look at her. Look back at her face, say "God, you're gorgeous," then kiss your way down from her tummy to her thighs.

– **Assuming you've done lots of finger foreplay** (see page 82), she should be open. If her labia lips are closed, use your nose to do the job. It also lets her know you aren't put off by her smell or secretions.

– **Consciously relax** your tongue, and your neck and facial muscles. It will stop you getting stiff and will feel better her end. Don't tense your tongue and make it pointy, relax it so it's wide and soft and can cover a larger area.

Imagine you're having a threesome with Angelina Jolie, Pamela Anderson, and the hot girl you see on the train every morning. Or the hot guy. Do whatever it takes to eke that final little bit more out of that weary, weary tongue.

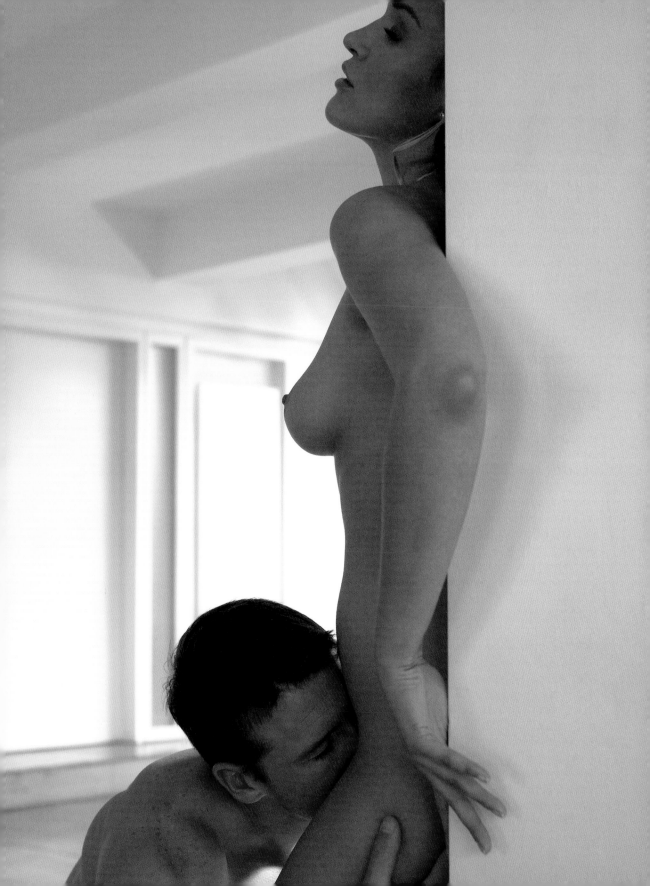

- **Make sure you've got plenty of saliva** in your mouth so your tongue's slippery rather than sandpapery, then lay it flat in between the lips of her labia, swishing it ever-so-gently to provide soft but pulsating pressure. The whole of your mouth will be against her (remember what I said about forgetting what you've seen in the porn movies?).

- **Be constantly aware of her body language.** If she lets out a little cry when you first stimulate her clitoris, it's not necessarily a good sign. It can be a cry of pain. What's your tongue doing? Really strong licking with a tensed tongue feels bloody awful. Some women like their clitoris sucked, like they do in porn movies, but most hate it! Give it up and try a gentler technique.

- **While the clitoris is definitely the star of the show,** don't focus exclusively on it to begin with. Try stiffening your tongue and pushing it inside her like a pretend penis or swirling it in circles just a little way in (most of the nerves are in the first inch anyway). Take a break to move up and lick her breasts, bite her neck, stroke and lick her thighs, the area between her anus and vagina, or try rimming (licking around her anus). Then get back to work on the little man in the boat, trying any or all of the following: long licks with the flat of your tongue, a fluttering side-to-side motion, circles, and zig-zags. Mix it up by using combinations of fast, slow, soft, and firmer (note I said "firmer" not hard) techniques.

- **Lick, don't flick.** You'll probably find she likes licking more than flicking. "I hate it when they flick it" was one of the most common responses I got when asking girls which oral techniques they did and didn't like.

- **A really simple way to find her hottest spot** is to trace a figure-eight with your tongue or lick all the letters of the alphabet (lower case is better because the letters are curlier). Both techniques stop any one part of the clitoris from being overstimulated. It's also great tongue-training. Practice on your palm—bet your tongue hurts before you get to *mmmmm*.

- **Just like with intercourse, most women end up settling on two or three favorite strokes,** with one as the guaranteed-to-get-me-there. The time to find this out is at the beginning, change techniques as she's about to come and she'll never, ever (ever) forgive you.

Can't find her clitoris?

If you're having trouble finding her clitoris, she might not be ready for you to! It will swell and become obvious once she's aroused.

- If it's still not obvious then say, "Show me where it feels good to you," rather than "I can't find your clitoris," and you won't feel like you're the dunce of Sex School. You're looking at the top end of her vagina for a teensy-weensy marble that could be tucked inside a hood of skin.

- When it's aroused, the clitoris usually comes out. If it doesn't, lick the hood gently or put the tip of your tongue on the hood and move it in circles, using it as a "buffer" like you would a foreskin. If it doesn't emerge but she's pulling you closer, place the heel of your palm on her pubic mound (the fleshy bit), fingers pointed to her belly and push toward her tummy. This exposes her clitoris.

- Gently lick around the sides, make circles around it, or lap at the bottom. Don't lick directly on it and remember: wide tongue, wet, gentle, slow, slow, slow. (Did I mention go slow?)

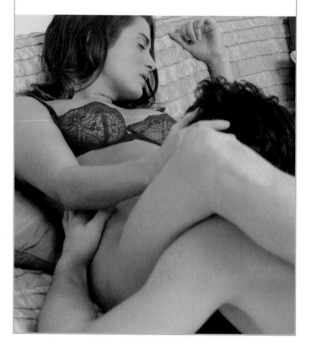

Ask her to tell you how each technique feels as you're trying it out. If she's too shy to say "That feels great" or "I don't like that one," tell her to grip the top of your arms if she likes it. The harder she grips, the more she likes it. (A few bruises never hurt anyone.)

– **When you know her favorite place to be licked,** tease her in another session by going close to it but not *quite* there. Occasionally move your tongue to where she wants it. It's cruel—and she'll get annoyed if you do it too long—but also hot as hell if you want to get her to begging point. (Or want to get out of doing the dishes.)

– **Starting to wonder if it's ever going to happen ...** and it's only been five minutes? Dear, oh dear, did they teach you nothing in school? (Sorry, I forgot—they don't! Most countries have an appalling sex education system.) It's probably going to take a lot longer than that, my lovely, so settle in. While you might take an average of four minutes to orgasm, she can do the same if she's super turned-on but might also take up to 15–20 minutes. Help her get there faster by …

– **Adding fingers.** Either thrust your fingers inside her or make a "V" with your index and middle finger and slide them back and forth with the clitoris in between, as you continue licking. Or get her to put her fingers inside herself while you lick. Reach up and squeeze her breasts.

– **Resist the urge to go faster** in an attempt to get her to orgasm quicker. If anything, slow down. The gentler and slower and more consistent you are, the quicker she'll get there. (Though it's not a race to get to the finish line even if that is where the "intercourse" flag tantalizingly waves.)

– **If she's not even close but you're so tired** you're losing the will to live, do one of two things. Either reach down and grab the small vibe you've put beside the bed for that purpose and hold it close to the clitoris as you continue to lick (or kiss her instead and just let the vibe do its stuff). Or simply ask her if she wants to stop and/or move on to something else.

– **She might not be able to get there** for a myriad of reasons that have nothing to do with the technique you're using (she's got work problems on her mind,

Remember, be gentle, slow, and consistent when giving her oral. It's not a race to the finish even if that's where the "intercourse" flag tantalizingly waves.

her ex called that morning, it's raining, the cat's just jumped on the bed)—and she's likely to be as fed up and frustrated about this as you are.

– **If she seems close but your attention is wavering** and your tongue's tired, the advice is completely different. I don't care what it takes but do NOT stop! Imagine you'll win a million dollars if you just keep going that little bit longer. Imagine you're having a threesome with Angelina Jolie, Pamela Anderson, and the hot girl you see on the train every morning. Or the hot guy. Do whatever it takes to eke that final little bit more out of that weary, weary tongue. And if you honestly can't keep moving it, just press it firmly and let her move against you for a few seconds, licking again the second you recover. (Don't change techniques, go straight back to what you were doing.) Continue throughout her orgasm (perhaps upping the speed and pressure a little just before it) and—crucially—do not stop until she pushes you away. Her orgasm lasts way, way longer than yours does.

– **Some women love you to immediately penetrate** the second it's over, while they're still riding the waves. If you do, you can set off a further set of scrumptious contractions. Others need time to recuperate and want to lie there panting for a bit. The good news is, she won't do what you do and roll over and go to sleep. Her body doesn't release the sleep hormone yours does, to get her ready for another round. Most of us can keep going without a recharge. Though chocolate and a glass of bubbly wouldn't go amiss in the breaks.

If she doesn't want you to give her oral, or you're not keen yourself, see page 182 for advice.

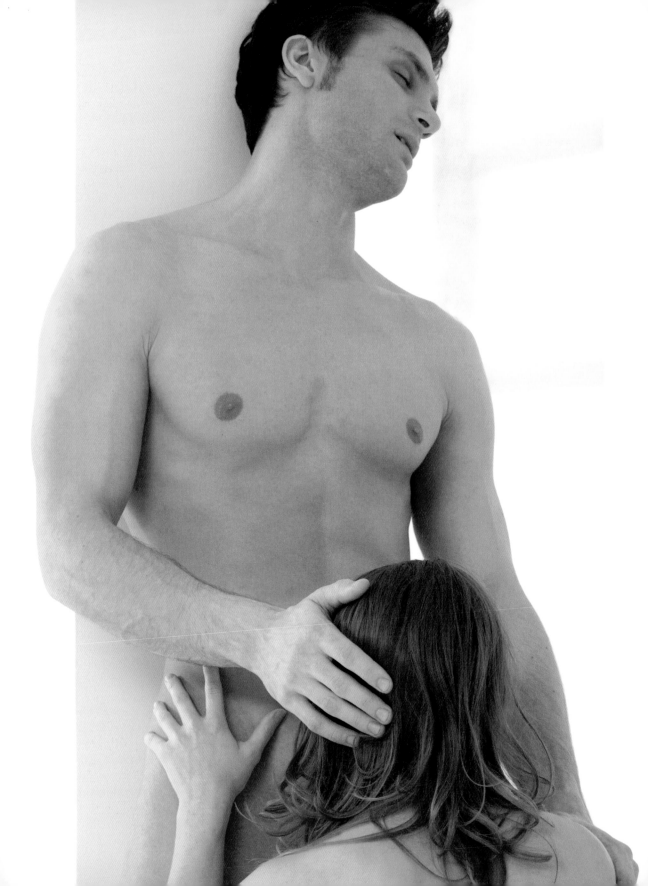

Giving him oral

Pick your position

– **He takes ages.** He stands, legs spread and with a wall behind him in case he wants to lean as things heat up. You kneel on some pillows before him. It's the classic porn pose so he'll have masturbated to it many times, speeding up the orgasm. You also appear to be worshiping the part he clearly does as well. Hot it up further by doing it completely naked while he's clothed (albeit pants unzipped). Or he's naked and you're completely clothed. This also allows good access to his scrotum, perineum, and anus—and stimulating any or all of these will push him over the edge.

– **He takes over.** Tie him up so he has no choice but to let you be the boss. Just as bondage works for you because it forces you to give up that "good girls shouldn't" attitude, it allows him to let go of the "I should be the one doing everything to her" attitude. You're in control, which also means no pushing of heads or him thrusting in your mouth.

– **He's shy.** Bless! Get him to kneel on the bed, at the headboard end with his back to the wall. You spread out face-down and any self-consciousness will disappear as he's treated to the view of your back, bottom, and legs before him. A traditional you-or-him-on-top 69er (see page 121) is also worth a try because there's no chance of eye contact.

– **He's begging for it.** Get primal. He lies on his back on the bed and you spread his arms and legs. You then straddle him, facing his feet. Use your feet to pin down his wrists and put your hands on his thighs, for support and to play dominatrix. You'll only have your tongue free but he'll be that turned on, it'll be all you need.

– **You want to impress.** Do it in semi-public, even if just for 10 precious seconds. A bit of playful exhibitionism gets instant admiration (it can also get you arrested, so take calculated risks). If you really, really want to score points, lie back on the bed with your head hanging over the edge of the bed. This is the position women use to "deep throat." The idea is to align your throat so it's in one long straight line then concentrate on completely relaxing the muscles. Inhale through your nose as he enters your mouth. Exhale as you slide him in deep.

If you get the urge to gag, swallow and it should disappear. (Practice on a carrot or dildo first.) Now, we all know deep throating—taking him as far as possible into your mouth—is a gimmick. (Most of the nerves are in the head, not the shaft.) But it's very porny and makes you appear utterly uninhibited and terribly experienced. If, indeed, this is the impression you want to give. If not stick to the public unzip and dip instead.

Take him to heaven

– **Start licking before you take his pants down.** Through his jeans (yes, really—with a *really* firm tongue) and then his underwear. Use the flat of your tongue against his Calvins, slithering the fabric around the shaft.

– **Even if he's already aroused,** don't grab his penis like it's the controller of your new game console. Lick your way there, bypass the goodies, back up the inner thigh, then lightly stroke his testicles and try out some hand techniques (see page 83).

– **Choose your position carefully,** especially if it's the first time, because you'll definitely want to use two hands and be comfortable. One should nearly always be around the shaft or you'll both have that funny but undignified "bobbing for apples" situation where you're chasing his penis all over the place.

– **If you're a naughty girl** (and if you aren't, why not?), you'll have already scooped a little pre-ejaculatory fluid (the white stuff that comes out the top, pre-orgasm), rubbed it on your lips, then kissed him. If you haven't, do it now or put your fingers inside yourself and use your own natural lubricant to lubricate him.

You can misjudge and play orgasm yo-yo so much, his penis just says "Screw it" and gives up. Bring him to the brink and back a few times, not 10.

The basic technique

Grip him at the base—this keeps the blood in the penis and keeps him nice and hard—then put your lips over the head and form a seal.

– You want slight suction so there's pressure but you don't literally suck.

– Press the flat of your tongue against his frenulum and wiggle experimentally. Then move into the hand follows mouth routine, slipping a loose fist up and down following the movement of your mouth so he can't tell the difference between your mouth and your hand.

– Your fist closes as you come to the head and opens as you travel down the shaft, getting firmer as he does, or the quicker you want him to orgasm. If he prefers you not to use your hand, use it to stabilize him at the base but don't slide it up and over.

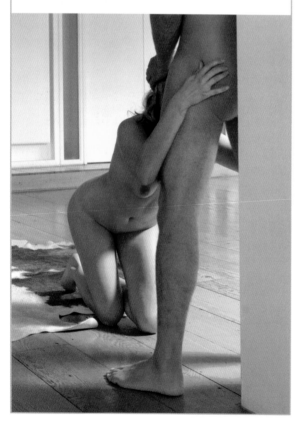

– **Make eye contact or tell him to watch you.** Make sure he can see the action by leaving the lights on, doing it in daylight, and either tying your hair back or getting him to hold it back.

– **Think about the big, first moment beforehand.** Either dispense long, lollipop licks (again holding the base). Or take just the velvety smooth head in your mouth. Or lean over and take the whole of him inside in one, smooth, practiced movement.

– **Don't stretch your lips over your teeth.** You'll look weird, and it's easier and more comfortable to push your lips forward, remaining diligently conscious of keeping your teeth out of the way. Now move into the basic technique (see left). Work into a nice rhythm, breathing through your nose (obviously).

– **Deal with the gagging thing** by always being in a position to control how deep he goes. If he puts his hands on the back of your head and pushes himself in to an uncomfortable point, stop completely, look him in the eye, and say "I don't like it when you do that. You won't do that again, will you?" (You might want to remove him from your mouth first for a sterner effect!) Don't continue until he reassures you. If your gag reflex is still strong even if he's not in terribly far, aim so he's hitting the roof of your mouth or side of your cheek. It can also feel quite nice if you push his penis against the hard palate on the roof of your mouth, letting it slide across the ridged surface.

– **Lick his perineum**—the smooth, hairless bit between his bottom and testicles—but first tell him how you're going to pretend it's another woman's vagina and this is what you'd do if you were in a threesome. (Yes, his hopes will be dashed when you reveal afterward that it remains just a fantasy. But it works well at the time.)

– **Let him play with you while you're playing with him.** Letting him see his fingers disappear inside you while his penis disappears into your mouth is one of life's best moments. Research shows his stimulation levels rise when he's playing with your body while receiving stimulation. Another trick: let him suck on your fingers as you suck him. It's not just sexy, most guys will suck your fingers the way they want you to suck them. So you'll pick up vital clues. Sneakily.

- **Move back to the frenulum**. Hold the base firmly, then delicately flick it using the flat of your tongue, using a steady pulsing motion. Try fluttering. Alternate with swirls around the corona. Try sucking it between your lips, *not* teeth, and playing with it. Suck it gently, roll it, use your other hand to play with the bottom of the shaft and gently knead the testicles.

- **It's a little boring** to concentrate *only* on the head and frenulum, and it can become desensitized or even painful. Move to the testicles, taking one into your mouth, one at a time and sucking lightly. Press your fingers on his perineum. Flutter a hard tongue back and forth across or inside the slit in the head. (He'll either love or hate this, so be warned.)

- **If you're doing your job properly,** he should be having a very nice time. Like eyeballs rolling back in head good time. Which should, in turn, get you off. Being able to wield this much power, reduce those powerful legs to jelly, make him *beg* for you to keep going ... My God girl, the power trip alone is enough to make you molten. (I remain convinced in my theory that women who don't like giving him oral—and men who don't like doing it to her—don't really like sex. Or they're gay.) And if you're enjoying giving him this much pleasure, let him know. Moan. Make noise. Stop (but not if he's on the edge), pull back, look at him and say "This is such a turn-on." Or simply, "God," then get your mouth back there.

- **While it's good to bring him to the brink of orgasm,** then slow it right down again (he's no different to you—the longer he takes to get there, the more intense it usually is), he's also like you in the sense that you can misjudge and play orgasm yo-yo so much, his penis just says "Screw it" and gives up. So bring him to the brink a few times, rather than 10.

- **If you've got the opposite problem** and he's looking cool as a cucumber, while you're breaking into a sweat from the exertion, you might need to ask him what he needs. Some guys orgasm quickly and *hard* through a head-job. Others find the sensation more subtle than intercourse. Use a strong hand grip and make sure you're adding the twist with your hand when you reach the head and a simultaneous swirl with your tongue. If that doesn't work, try inserting a well-lubed finger to stimulate the prostate (put a finger up his butt, in other words). Or stimulate other sensitive parts externally by using the side of your hand and pressing it really hard, in between his legs on the perineum.

- **Think *way* before he orgasms,** what you're going to do—as in swallow or not swallow—rather than dither around and botch the whole thing. There's lots of practical tips for dealing with this on page 120, but your basic choices are to swallow, remove your mouth and let him ejaculate elsewhere, or hold it in your mouth and spit it out afterward. The last one is the least favorite option because it somehow implies you're repulsed by his sperm. How would you feel if he bolted to the sink after licking you to rinse out his mouth? Exactly.

What's hot

Always keep it wet, lick *hard* rather than too soft and, remember, as a general rule, the bigger the penis, the harder the pressure you should use. The more your tongue moves, the better. Swirl it around the head, lick up and down the shaft, push it under and around the rim, lap at the base.

What's not

Freezing cold hands are almost as scary as long fingernails but not as bad as scratchy ones that have ragged cuticles. Jagged teeth, rings with stones protruding out of threatening metal claws, yanking back the foreskin rather than coaxing ... don't be guilty of any of them. And don't assume what Henry loved, Harry will too.

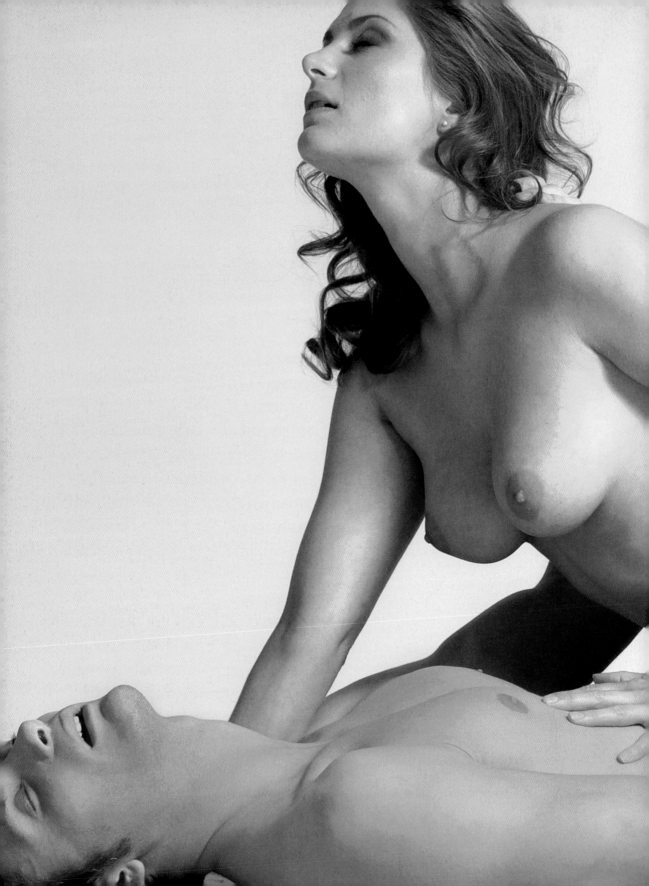

Destination Orgasm

If sex is the journey, then orgasm is surely the place we've all bought tickets for. Find out the best route, enjoy the local hotspots—and guarantee many return visits!

Is sex all about having an orgasm? If it is all about that 30-second (if you're very, very lucky) rush of euphoria, we'd all hurry to get there, surely? Women would rush home to their vibrators—the most reliable, quickest way to climax for her—and men would hurry home to watch internet porn—fast becoming the most reliable, quickest route for him. Instead, we make a supremely valiant effort to have sex with each other, in various combinations (depending on if you're gay, straight, or bi), but still with the same result—a far less reliable way to get our rocks off. It's much easier to achieve a DIY orgasm than have one with another human being. For a start, your thoughts are much easier to control when you're alone.

I once had a potentially excellent orgasm completely ruined because the person who was giving it to me kept morphing into Gollum. For the one person in the world who hasn't seen Lord of the Rings, Gollum is a slimy, super-skinny computer-generated creature with disproportionately large hands and feet. Not the sort you want to be sleeping with (obviously). The guy I was with when the film came out was a bit on the lean side, with incredibly slim hips and quite a large penis. I found it oddly disturbing—like the wrong body part had been attached to the wrong person. Just like Gollum's too- large hands and feet ... And the second my brain made the association, the relationship was doomed.

One minute my skinny (but handsome) boyfriend was between my legs, delivering what was actually damn good oral sex, the next Gollum was looking up at me with those bulging eyes hissing "My precious." Over. Both the potential orgasm and (sadly, bless him) the relationship.

But did this send me scuttling to solo sex, vowing never to do it any other way? Of course not. Because it's real-life relationships that add the sizzle to any orgasm. The tummy flip-flops you get before a date, analyzing who said what when and what it all means afterward, sneaking secret glances at their bits, longing to kiss, touch, lick, and bite them, feeling squirmy and wet or hard and achy—masturbation orgasms during this stage are at their most intense, fueled by anticipation of what's surely to (dear God) come soon. Then there's the very first time they touch us, lick us, penetrate—even more shivery, spectacular fantasy fodder to fuel our orgasms, whether still solo or not. If love gets added to the equation, there's skin contact, pumping hormones, snuggling, eye-gazing—they all pile up on top to fast-track us into orgasms unlike any we'd experience alone.

There's a reason why we jump through extraordinarily complicated hoops to not only make someone like us but lust after us—it might be harder to have an orgasm with another person but it's usually a far superior quality. And that goes for both men and women. There's a perception that because men's orgasms are easier to come by, quality isn't important. It is. His orgasms differ in quality just as hers do. My aim here is to make it easier to orgasm with each other and to make those orgasms good. Very, very good. I'll start with ways to vamp up both your orgasm quotas, move on to a treat for him, then one for her too!

Call them anal, oral, G-spot, clitoral, multiple, sequential, or whatever the hell you like, but there's still only one type of orgasm.

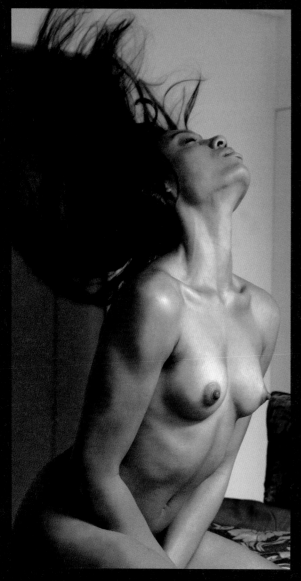

An orgasm is an orgasm!

Anatomically, all orgasms come from the same place even if some feel different than others. There is only one physical type of orgasm for both men and women, no matter how much we try to pretend there are more. Call them anal, oral, G-spot, clitoral, multiple, sequential, or whatever the hell you like, but an orgasm is still simply our body releasing blood back into the bloodstream after it's been pumped to pressure point to an aroused area. Whether you got to that point through oral sex, vaginal sex, anal play, using a vibrator, or eating spaghetti while standing on your head, the mechanics are the same. It's crucial for you both to understand this if you want more orgasms yourself and for your partner.

But what's also essential to understand is that while the process might always be the same, the feeling registered in the brain isn't. Some orgasms are weak, pathetic little pulses, others strong and mighty. What makes the difference? Emotion, erotic desire, experimentation, skill, timing, patience, chemistry, love—any and all can do it.

I want orgasms that are ...

More frequent

– **You want a quickie.** Using lots of lube, he holds a vibrator against her clitoris and penetrates from behind. Egos are less important than orgasms in this scenario.

– **You'd rather be having sex with someone else.** Pretend that you are. Your partner can't read your mind. If you don't tell them, how are they supposed to know? Quit the guilt trip—almost all men and women admit to fantasizing about someone else while with a (still much-loved) partner. Sex with someone else is OK in your head, it's only bad if it's in your bed.

– **You missed out on one during intercourse.** Masturbate afterward while your partner watches. Take a really long time if they didn't try hard enough to make you orgasm during it.

– **You want to experiment but feel self-conscious.** Try blindfolding your partner—you'll feel less inhibited if there's no eye contact and be more inclined to let go and enjoy it. Plus it means they can't see the bits where it all goes a bit wonky.

You can't quite get there. Be super-alert for your personal orgasm triggers. The more your brain travels a certain path neurologically, the more effortless it becomes. The more signposts of impending orgasm your brain can recognize, the easier it will trigger the orgasmic response. Focus on what you naturally do on approach to orgasm, then exaggerate it. If that doesn't work, take the pressure off by giving up completely. Better luck next time.

You're doing it missionary style. The traditional "jackhammer" style of thrusting—a deep, repetitive in-and-out motion—is about as effective at getting her to orgasm as using a bread knife to shave your legs. Instead, try her grinding against his pelvis and move in circles, rather than up and down. The aim is to keep as much of the base of his penis as possible in contact with the whole of the vulva. He should keep thrusting short and shallow rather than deep and fast.

You're doing it standing up. If you're standing up having sex at least one of you felt a spontaneous, urgent need. This lends itself nicely to roleplaying or talking dirty. If you just went along with it to be nice, be nice about indulging this as well.

You're doing it doggy style. She can lift her bottom high so he's hitting the super-sensitive front vaginal wall, he reaches forward to play with her clitoris before he's fully penetrated, she reaches behind to play with his testicles. Choose opposite sides to reach from.

He's on top. Spread her vaginal lips once he's inside and make sure they're pressed against him to get maximum friction on the clitoris and the area around the urethra. It's also packed with nerve endings. Spark memories of the great oral you just had by licking and sucking each other's tongues. Try not to dribble ...

She's on top. This is the most likely position to result in orgasms-for-two because she can slow things down if he starts to lose it. If you're trying to come together, he should be alert to a tightening of her vagina. When she's around a level 8 on a 1–10 pleasure scale, her vagina will often grip his penis tighter. The biological purpose is to make him orgasm so he'll spill his seed but it's OK to use for less worthy purposes, like an "OK, we're about to lift off" signal.

Rev up for round two (three, four, five ...).

There are four different types of multiple orgasms.

– Compounded single orgasms: each one is distinct and separate but there's more than one in the same session.

– Sequential: these multiple orgasms happen fairly close together in that you don't stop to watch TV or take a shower and the level of arousal stays fairly constant.

– Serial: mere seconds separate your orgasms with no real interruption between them and no let up in stimulation (how many bowls of Wheaties did you have this morning?).

– Blended: a mix of two or more of the above.

Are you exhausted just hearing about these options? Once can be enough. Otherwise, try aiming for compounded singles—just more than one orgasm per session.

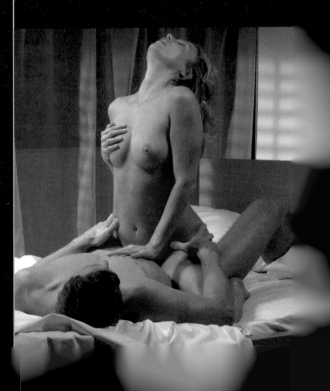

It's much easier to achieve a DIY orgasm than have one with another human being. For a start, your thoughts are much easier to control when you're alone.

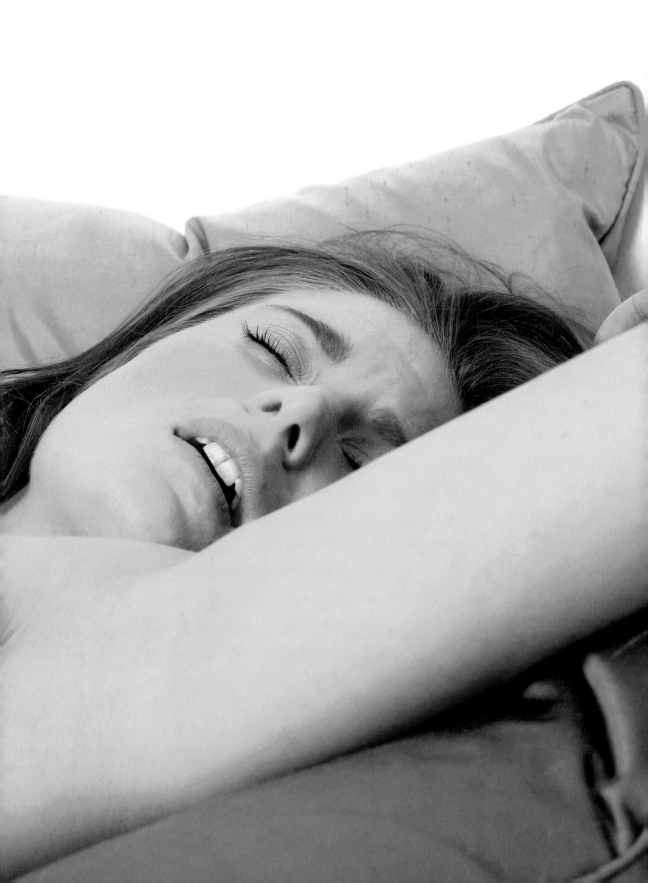

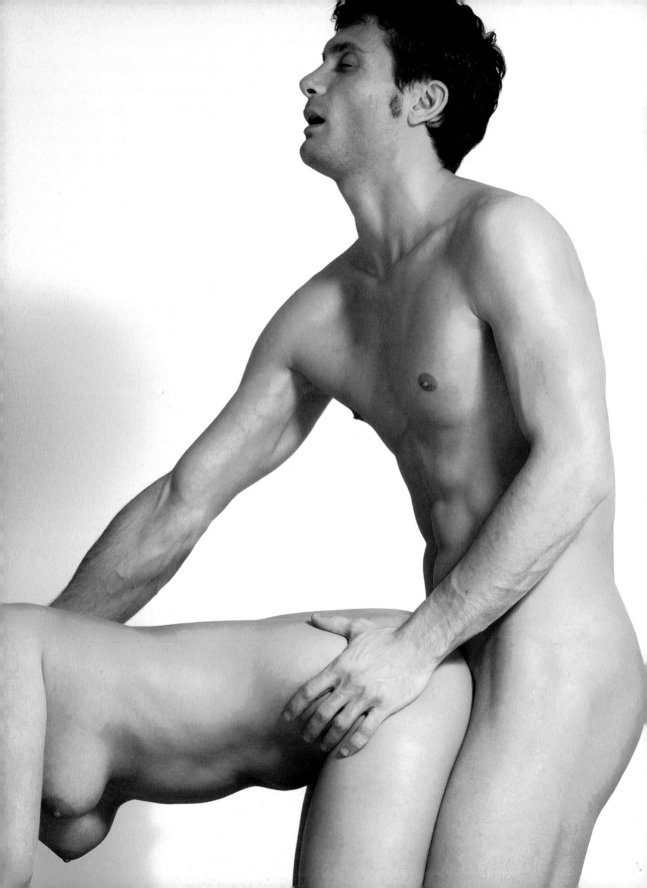

1

If you're distracted, keep your eyes open and watch the action instead of losing yourself in "Wonder what Jenny/John really meant when they said that?".

2

For a more intense sex session, try to stay focused on what you're feeling to distract yourself from what you're thinking. Stay in the moment.

3

Get your partner to stimulate two spots at once. He can insert a well-lubed thumb into her bottom while licking her. She can reciprocate when giving him oral.

4

Choose a new, challenging position for intercourse. This will force you to concentrate and stay in the moment. Balance or die.

More intense

- **Don't be drunk.** It relaxes inhibitions but is likely to numb other parts too.

- **Aim for sequential orgasms.** Not simultaneous. You'll have stronger orgasms if you're focused on your own pleasure rather than trying to work out where your partner is on the arousal scale. Coming together is awfully polite but the pay-off can be fizzlers and failure.

- **Pee first.** Nothing worse than the whole "Is this an orgasm or do I just want to wee?" thing—especially if you're trying G-spot stimulation (see pages 58–63).

Multiple

- **Lower your expectations if you're a man.** This is the pay-off for women. It's hard for us to have an orgasm but once we do, it's easier to have more. Men learn to have multiple orgasms by learning techniques. Women are just engineered for them.

- **Train yourself through masturbation.** Masturbate in your usual way until you're almost, almost ... then stop. Change to a new position, switch to a different technique (for example, ditch the vibe and use fingers instead), then start again. Again get almost there then stop. Change position and technique again—and keep doing it till you've brought yourself to the brink at least five times. This technique not only stops your body from expecting exactly the same stimulation to orgasm, it trains it to expect that after one peak of sensation, another is coming.

- **Use different types of stimulation.** Alternate oral sex with intercourse with digital stimulation (that's fingers rather than digital TV, but while we're on the topic, a bit of porn playing in the background could be just what you need to add another to the list!).

- **Other ways to make it happen.** *Simmer* by anticipating what's in store, way before you touch them. *Be* in the right head space to keep going. *Avoid* small, sensitive areas immediately after the first orgasm. The nerve endings are too on edge so instead zoom in on larger hot spots like breasts, bottom cheeks, inner thighs, backs. *Kiss* with tongues fighting like gladiators. *Rub* your bodies together during intercourse and maintain full body contact. *Pump* those pelvic floor muscles. *Add* erotic edge by pulling her hair, spanking his butt.

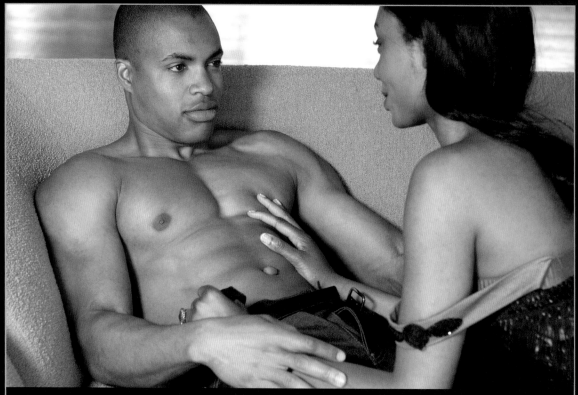

To make his better

Yes, we all know the joke says simply handing him a beer and taking off your clothes will get a result. But we're after a *gobsmacker* of an orgasm here, so start with the beer and nakedness and add a whispered promise that he doesn't have to do anything, just *take*. Believe me, he's in heaven already.

– Ask him to masturbate while you watch. Especially watch where he first places his hand at the start— that's exactly where you place yours when you take over the hand-job. (It may sound unimportant but it's the key to accurately mimicking the motion.)

– Pay attention to how firm and fast his grip is. If he's practically strangling the thing without wincing, your best bet to deliver an earth-shattering orgasm probably isn't through intercourse. Do your pelvic floor exercises all you like but unless your day job is shooting out ping-pong balls in a sex bar, it's unlikely your vagina will rival the grip of a tightly closed fist that's yanking fiercely.

– If that's how he did it, do him in reverse. Start with intercourse—jump on top and let him penetrate for a few, short, exquisite minutes while you pump your pelvic muscles around him—then jump off and finish him off, using your hand (gripping hard) and mouth together. If his grip wasn't too hard, fellate him, then jump on top to let him penetrate. Don't bounce, instead rock back and forth, rubbing your clitoris against his pelvis.

– Most guys have one particular "added extra" that really does it for them. It might be ball play, a finger inserted up his bottom, tweaking or biting a nipple, hearing you talk dirty, watching porn, being tied up ... If he won't tell you, try the lot (perhaps not all in one go) and see which he most responds to.

– The longer the build-up, the better the orgasm so tease mercilessly and don't forget to moan when he climaxes to show him it's a turn-on for you. Award yourself a gold star if you can make yourself orgasm at the same time as you're letting him take, take, take (guilt-free), simply by humping his leg.

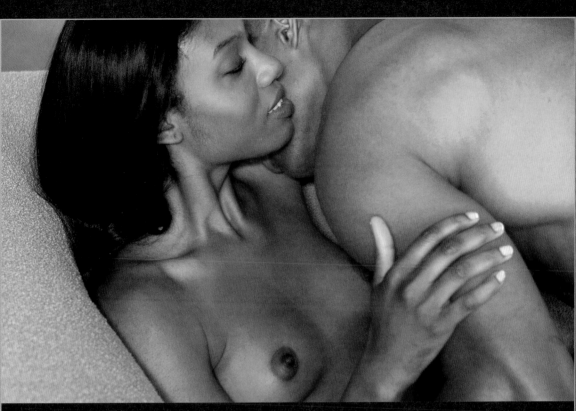

To make hers better

So if passing you a beer and getting naked whets your whistle, what does it for her? Try turning up with a champagne and chocolate-dipped strawberries combo (or even plain old ordinary ones if you've left it to the last minute). It reminds us of the scene in *Pretty Woman* and adds a dash of sophistication even if you are still wearing your softball gear.

– Nothing turns us on more than our bodies being admired—with your eyes, with trailing fingertips, your touches becoming less restrained when you finally get your hands on the top half. There is nothing sexier than watching someone's eyes change as lust rudely elbows desire out of the way—let her see this.

– Undress her, stay dressed yourself. Kiss and lick through her underwear—tease through it, push it to one side, play. Before removing her bra, kiss her neck and grab a handful of her hair and pull it, just a little, make eye contact then deliver a deep long kiss.

– Massage her breasts, kiss her neck again then move south, pooling saliva in your mouth as you go, so the first lick on her vulva will be soft and *slippery*. Smell her, moan, then move into swishing and licking (see pages 40–43). Push a finger inside her, then two. Turn her over and pushing your hand through her legs, keep gently rubbing her clitoris and lick around her anus. If she pulls away, stroke her bottom while you're playing with her clitoris, kiss her neck and then turn her over again.

– Choose an intercourse position. Take her from behind if she seems to crave an animal approach. When her breathing becomes ragged, add lube, and use your fingers to slide up and down between her labia, grazing her clitoris while you thrust. If this all seems a bit too racy, opt for a spoons position from behind.

– Stop before you're too close to coming, and go back to licking her until she orgasms, then when she's at the tail end (wait at least 15 seconds), pull back and penetrate again, hopefully pushing her into another climax. Then, and only then, can you let go.

Gushing Over The G-Spot

Even though it's been 64 years since the original study, the world remains fascinated by what was once touted to be a "magic orgasm button". So ... is it? Let's find out.

Writing about the G-spot is a bit like hearing bell bottoms are coming back in fashion. Like, I was there the first time around. The original experiment that prompted the infamous book *The G-Spot* was carried out 64 years ago! No, I'm not that old but when the book was published in 1982, I remember *Cosmopolitan's* coverline announcing a "magic orgasm button." When I went to work in the editorial department at *Cosmo* four years later, we still had our panties in a frenzied knot over the G-spot. And here we are, over 20 years later, still arguing about it: is there or isn't there one? Can it make you ejaculate and, if so, how? Or isn't it really just an excuse because you accidentally let some pee out?!

Thankfully, the new G-spot theories make a hell of a lot more sense than the old ones. I've never disputed that the front vaginal wall has orgasmic potential—yes, I did once get there thanks to a man with an exceptional combination of long fingers, a long penis, and an equally long attention span—but I was just never convinced about the existence of something that was rumored to occur in some women's bodies but not others. Like, we've all got tonsils, hearts, and livers, so why would Mother Nature suddenly decide to randomly hand out another body part to some but not all? It's not logical. More recent research suggests everyone does have this "hot spot" but the amount of tissue and number of nerve endings varies from woman to woman. Which would explain why reaction to it ranges from massively enthusiastic to decidedly lukewarm.

Mention "G-spot" and you know the topic of "female ejaculation" isn't far behind. The reason why they sit so comfortably together is because stimulation of the G-spot is what seems to cause women to ejaculate. The spongy tissue around the urethra (see page 60) contains between 30–40 glands and ducts. These glands are thought to be responsible for producing the fluid females ejaculate. Give the G-spot what it likes and ejaculatory fluid is sometimes produced, flowing from the glands through the ducts into the urethra before escaping out of the body. Straight onto your newly washed sheets.

Whatever your thoughts on the G-spot, read on ... If nothing else, it will mean you're not completely clitoris-centered. Sure, your fingers are always going to go back there, but hey, nothing ventured ...

We've all got tonsils, hearts, and livers, so why would Mother Nature suddenly decide to randomly hand out a body part to some women but not all? It's not logical.

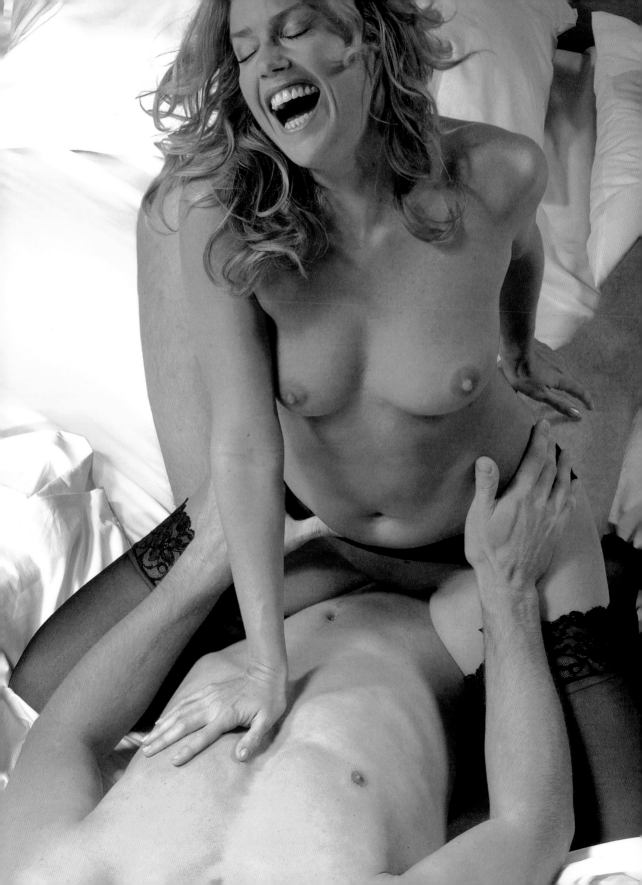

How to find your G-spot

It's not hard to find, it's just awkward. I'd suggest finding it yourself first, then guiding him.

- Get into position: if you're lying on your back, press your knees against your chest and then open them, or try squatting, or lying on your stomach. Some women find it easier to get on all fours and use one hand to prop themselves up.

- Slide your fingers inside, palm facing up, as if you're trying to touch your tummy, then hook them around slightly. Aim about 2–3 in (5–8 cm) inside and feel for slightly ridgy, textured tissue (it feels like the front of the roof of your mouth) on the front wall.

- Make a "come here" motion with your fingers, pulling them over the area.

- Pay attention to what you're feeling as well as what you're feeling for—don't focus exclusively on searching for ridges, also be alert to the places where it feels more sensitive. Experiment with different strokes and don't be scared to use firm, hard pressure—the G-spot's not as skittish as the touchy, tetchy clitoris.

- Keep going. The more aroused you are, the more the area will swell and the easier it will be to feel. Once you've found it, do some firm massaging.

- It's not surprising women tend to stick to clitoral orgasms during masturbation. To give yourself a G-spot orgasm, you have to twist your arm into a weird position and it's not exactly comfy. Which is where he comes in.

- Now you know where it is, he positions himself so he can reach it easily with his fingers. It's a lot easier for him to get to it than you but he still needs to hook his fingers around and aim for your tummy. Once he's found it, get him to add some oral for doubly delicious stimulation.

G-spot pleasure

So where is the G-spot?
Most people know their urethra—it's the tube you pee out of, right? Well there's spongy tissue wrapped around the urethra that's erectile—meaning it swells when blood fills it. Blood pumps into erectile tissue when we're aroused—it's just more obvious when it pumps into the cylinders of his penis because you can see it filling up.

Our erections aren't quite so visually spectacular, being hidden! This spongy, erectile area is the "urethral sponge" and the bit of the urethral sponge you can feel through the top wall of the vagina is, ladies and gentleman, the G-spot. (Well, it's the definition most people now seem to agree on anyway.) It's part of the same network of nerve endings that make up the hidden part of the clitoris, and it's also sometimes referred to as the female prostate (which makes sense, given the male prostate is the male "G-spot").

The cheat's way to enjoy a G-spot orgasm
This comes via specially designed vibrators. Gosh, why are we not surprised! The same device that delivers our most consistent and reliable clitoral orgasms, also works a treat on the G-spot.

- **G-spot vibrators** usually come with explicit instructions but it helps if you find the spot first with your finger (see box, left) then insert the vibrator.

- **The curved tip** of it points toward your top wall. Don't move it in and out of your vagina like you might a normal dildo or vibrator, instead make a rocking motion so it starts to feel like a firm massage.

- **If your vibrator has a ball** at each end, use one to roll it side to side once in position and hold the other one at the other end. If you like the sensation, try using your vibrator with him, while he's licking you. Don't be surprised if you need clitoral stimulation as well as G-spot to orgasm—it's not unusual.

- **Further intensify your orgasm** by either of you pressing down lightly on your lower abdomen while the vibrator is in there. This provides extra pressure on the "back side" of the G-spot (this also works during intercourse or when his fingers are inside you).

The need to pee!

When the sponge tissue swells, it presses against the urethra and bladder. A full bladder produces a similar sensation. You need to get past this feeling to orgasm, so if you're worried your bladder really is full, stop and go to the bathroom. Then go back to what you were doing. If the same sensation builds again, it's a pretty good bet you're on the verge of a G-spot orgasm and/or ejaculation. So how do they know it's not pee? Both ejaculate and urine come out of the same tube so there are bound to be traces of urine.

Also remember, the jury's still out on whether females ejaculate at all so there's not exactly a huge amount of research done on stuff like this. One much-cited experiment involved a lone woman who downed some medication designed to turn her urine blue, then embarked on a masturbatory session where she

Don't be scared to use quite firm or even hard pressure—the G-spot's not as skittish as the touchy, tetchy clitoris.

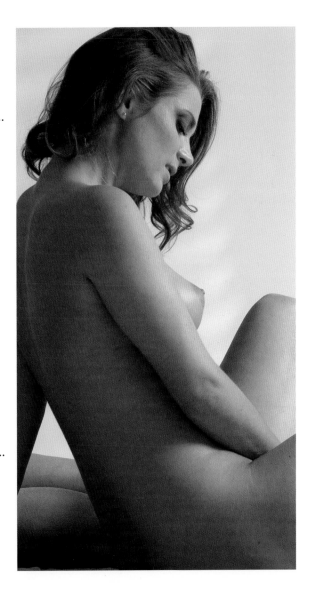

What's hot for him

The male G-spot is also near the urethra: it's the prostate gland. But while we can rummage around to find ours, his is a lot harder to get to. Find it for him by inserting a well-lubed finger into his anus, then feel up the front rectal wall until you find something that feels like a walnut. Hold your finger still until he relaxes, then start massaging firmly in a downward direction. It helps if he draws his knees up to his chest once you've found it.

What's not

Going there without warning him, or refusing to try. Not having trimmed nails. Touching your or his genitals afterward—it can spread bacteria.

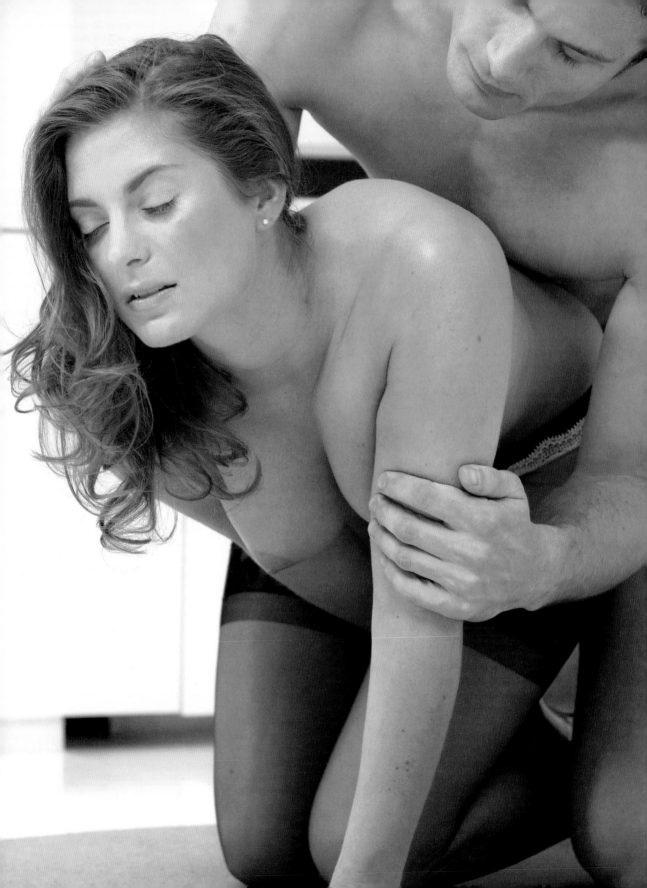

Clitoral or G-spot?

So is there much difference?

– A G-spot orgasm comes from the same nerve endings as a clitoral orgasm but the feeling appears to differ from woman to woman. Clitoral orgasms tend to feel more universal.

– You'd like the chance to find out the difference but the G-spot just isn't working for you? Unfortunately, unlike clitoral orgasms, which are more reliable, you can't guarantee you'll have a G-spot orgasm just because you've found your G-spot. Some women don't find it that sensitive. Others women find the opposite and find the sensation incredibly irritating because it's too intense. "It just feels like I'll die if I don't pee there and then, and I don't find that sexy at all," was the response of one girl who tried it.

– Most studies claim about two-thirds of women are sensitive to G-spot stimulation with probably one third really enjoying the experience. It's a bit like bottoms. People who love anal play tend to really love it. People who hate it, *really* hate it.

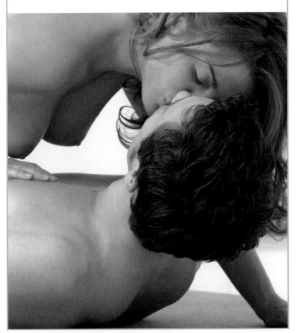

alternated between peeing and ejaculating on a sheet. She examined the color of each and said the pee came out dark blue and the ejaculate either clear or only slightly blue. Conclusive evidence? Who knows? No-one else was there and there was no control group—someone else just happened to report on it in a medical journal and because there's precious little info out there, everyone jumped on it. This often happens with sex research—huge presumptions based on such small samples. Women I've spoken to say the fluid they ejaculate is clear rather than yellow (or blue) and sometimes looks a bit milky. What little analysis has been done shows it to be made up of prostate-specific antigen (which is also present in semen).

Will you definitely ejaculate?
You might do. All women have the sponge but not all ejaculate. We do know you're more likely to ejaculate if you're incredibly aroused, that it's likely to be via G-spot stimulation, and that it helps if you've got strong pelvic floor muscles. Some women ejaculate a few measly little drops, others a cup or more. Most of the time, the women orgasm and ejaculate simultaneously but that's not always the case. So what's the difference between simply "getting wet" and ejaculating? Normal lubrication happens slower and more evenly. If you ejaculate, it tends to happen fast and usually around orgasm.

Can you teach yourself to ejaculate?
If you want to try, go for it. Do your kegels, use a G-spot vibrator, explore lots, and if you feel the urge to pee, don't hold it in. Devotees say it helps if you remove the toy (or finger or his penis) because that might stop the fluid gushing out. Of course, if you stop everything a little too hastily, the orgasm might disappear along with the hoped-for ejaculation, so timing's crucial! Like everything else sexual, G-spot orgasms are healthy to aim for, not so healthy to obsess about. There's no evidence that ejaculation makes for a better orgasm, by the way!

The G-spot's a bit like anal play. People who love it tend to really love it. People who hate it, *really* hate it.

Mission Possible

Given the simple but spectacular design screw-up that put her orgasm activator and his in totally different areas, can intercourse ever be equally pleasurable for both of you? Follow some new rules and you might just be pleasantly surprised ...

Here's why mutual intercourse orgasms aren't the norm. Her clitoris is *outside* her vagina, his penis goes *inside* her vagina during intercourse. This means the usual "pumping" style of thrusting does nothing to stimulate her most sensitive part. It is, however, a highly effective method to produce an orgasm for him. His most sensitive part, the frenulum, gets a nice, thorough seeing-to as it's rubbed up and down the vaginal walls. End result: happy man, not so happy woman.

But it's not all bad news. Lots of women love the feeling even if doesn't result in orgasm. The vaginal walls are sensitive, it feels good having you inside us, our G-spot actually *does* have a chance in hell of getting some action through intercourse and—thanks to lots of research devoted to solving the problem—there are now other techniques that help. This feature has a distinctly female-friendly slant but given the way the odds are stacked, that's sort of necessary don't you think? Having said that, you both should keep the following in mind:

You are allowed to take a break, you know. Sex is usually more effective if you move between penetrative sex, oral, kissing, using your hands, pee breaks, even little naps!

There's not a Commandment that says once you're having intercourse, you must keep going till at least one of you climaxes.

Desire fluctuates during a typical sex session. His erection will go up and down, her lubrication will wax and wane. Lube (see page 130) and a healthy hand-job (see pages 82–83) sorts both out.

Just because you start in one position, doesn't mean you have to stay in it. But don't go to the other extreme. Changing position to show off will have the opposite effect and show you up as being inexperienced.

It's usually easier to let her come first through clitoral-focused foreplay before moving on to intercourse, even though a practiced female-friendly thrusting style can make an enormous difference.

Compromise. The trouble with the "girl-grind" is that it tips the scale the opposite way. Grinding, full pelvis contact usually feels *way* better her end than his. Take turns indulging what feels best during the same session, or on different occasions. Give and take. Play nicely.

Move the mundane missionary to the bathroom floor and it becomes more primitive than killing a beast with your bare hands.

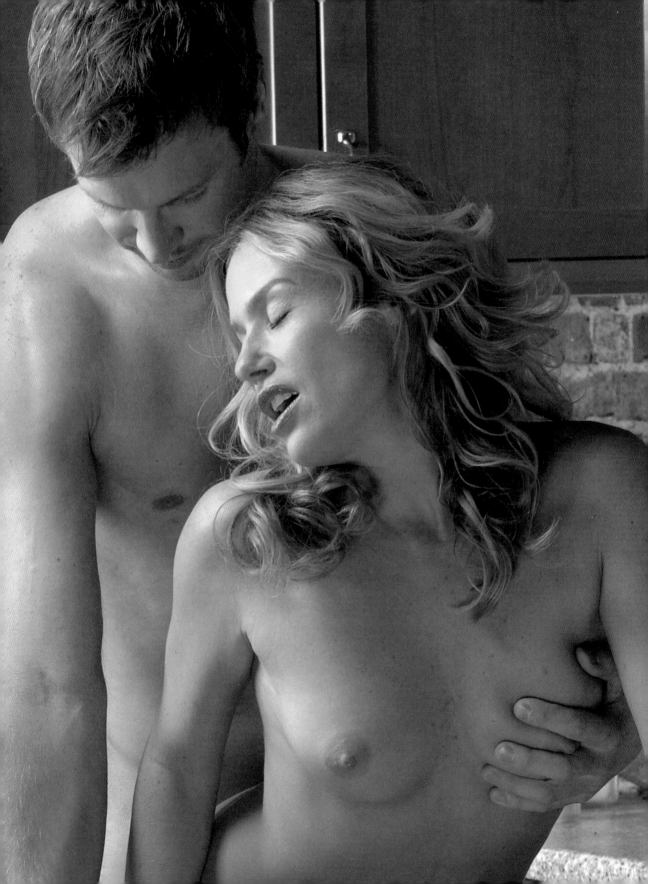

1

Doggy Does It

Doing it like they do on the Discovery Channel makes for detached sex (no eye contact means less guilt if you're cheating). But it's the anonymity and primal element that makes it so erotic, causing men to come quicker doing it doggy style than in other positions.

How quick? Well, 1.8 minutes to be precise (if he's really excited or suffers from PE). Which is exactly 5.5 minutes less than it takes for the average man to ejaculate with consistent rhythm. Yep, that's 7.3 minutes from the first thrust to the last. (Most guys think it's 15.) The average sexual "encounter," by the way, lasts 15–30 minutes. But whether we're talking a one-nighter or 10 years in, isn't made clear. The moral of this story: stop trying to live up to an "average" that doesn't exist. It's healthy for him to let loose and not spare the horses occasionally.

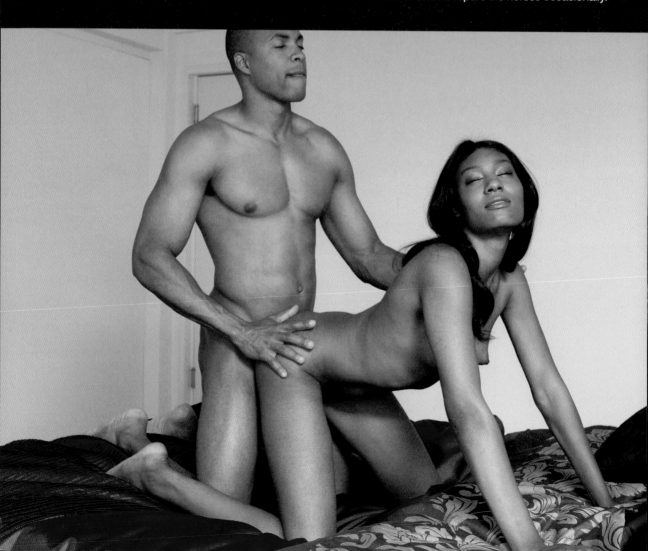

2 Cat Got Your Orgasms?

Switch to the CAT (Coital Alignment Technique) and you'll double her chances of climaxing—and slow him down by about the same rate. A winning combination! It's slightly harder work than the "pumping" style of thrusting and takes practice, but give it a try ...

He's on top of her but riding high, his body moved up toward her head and he's close rather than holding himself up on his arms. The pelvises are close, so the base of his penis rubs against her clitoris and *stays there* as they move together. Picture an even-paced rocking chair movement: she leads in the upward stroke, pushing up and forward to force his pelvis backward. He forces her pelvis backward and downward. It's pressure and counterpressure, not thrusting, with deep, not shallow, penetration.

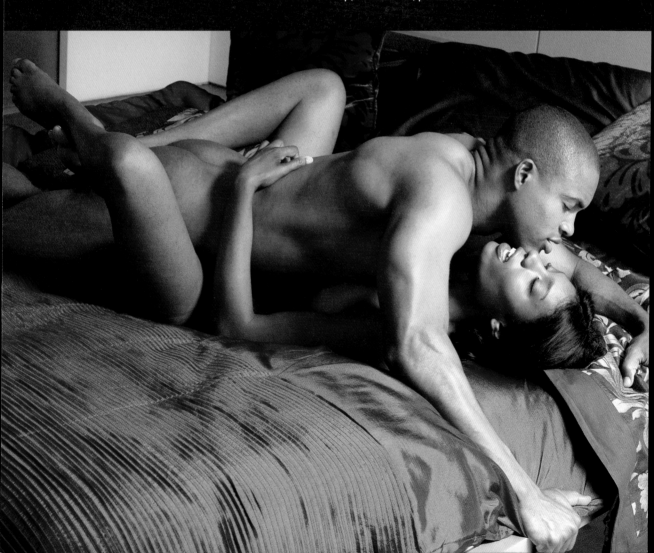

3
The Threesome That Works

Add a sex toy. This shows a classic vibe—versatile enough for most positions—but there are "no hands" alternatives. Vibrating penis rings are surprisingly efficient, as are wearable "butterfly" vibes (see page 139).

My favorite, though, is a new invention called a "We-Vibe." It's small, C-shaped, and she wears it during intercourse. Turn it on, insert one end up to the bend, and the whole thing opens to an "L" shape. The clitoral pad sits against the labia and clitoris, the other end works on the G-spot. It flattens out so smoothly, he can't feel it during sex but he does feel the powerful vibrations. It's causing quite a buzz (sorry), with men loving the sensation as much as women. I think it will become the way of the future. Even if this particular brand doesn't last, the design will.

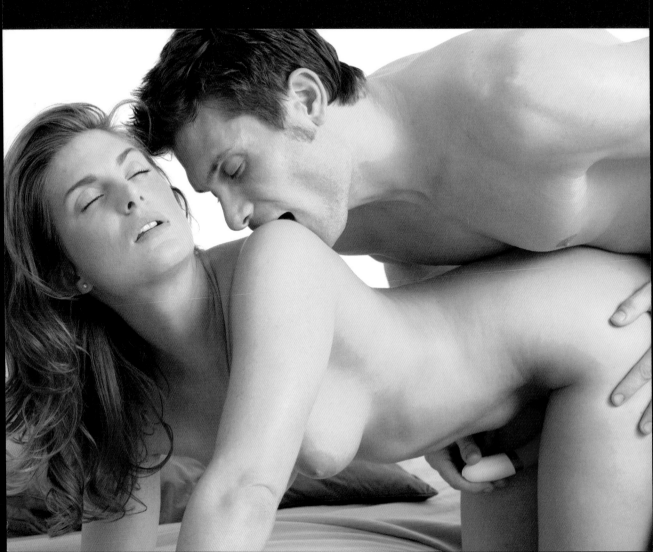

4
It Legging

Him on top nearly always makes a couple's top three positions because it's so versatile. Him kneeling instead of lying offers more range of movement, but it's the position of her legs that's vital for how this feels.

For deep penetration, she should put her legs on his shoulders—the higher and further back, the deeper his penis plunges. Spread her legs wide and make sure he's fully pressed against her pubic bone and lower abdomen for a magic tugging sensation on the clitoris. Keep her legs straight and together with his outside hers, for a tighter fit for him, while he grinds satisfyingly against her mons and clitoris. Most him-on-tops are improved by a pillow under her hips or bottom and he's better off using a rocking/grinding motion, unless it's *his* turn for a good old-fashioned pounding!

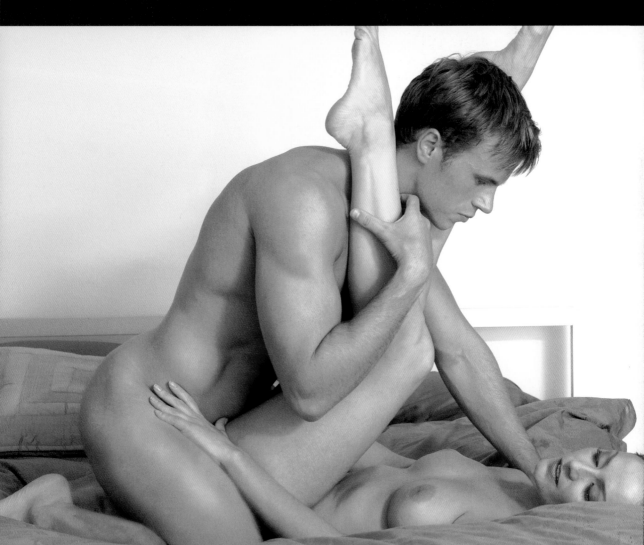

5
The V Technique

You'd be hard pressed to find a reputable sex expert who won't advise you to add clitoral stimulation to any and all intercourse positions. But who does the best job—him or her? She usually wins the prize, simply because most couples opt for stroking, which is hard for him to keep gentle and consistent while he's thrusting. His hand often gets knocked off target without him realizing—she can *feel* if it's all gone AWOL.

A technique that's easy for either of you is to make a V shape with the first two fingers of one hand (or whatever feels comfortable) and place them around the vagina so the penis slides in between. This stimulates the clitoris, inner labia, and urethra—as well as adding intensity for him. Or place the V either side of the clitoris, pushing your fingers down in a rocking rhythm.

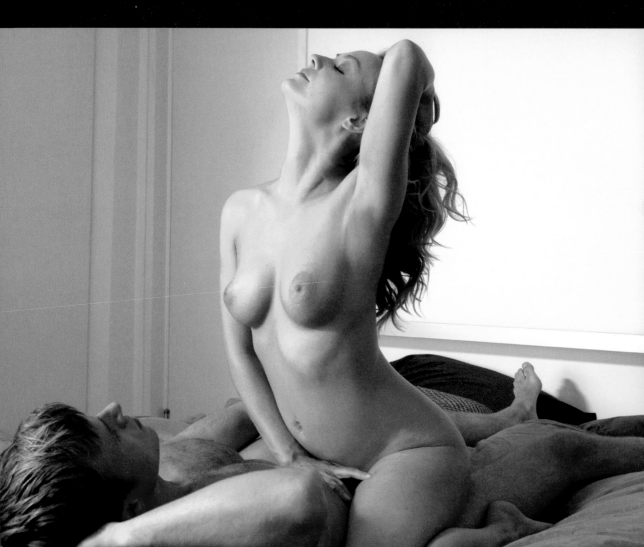

6

The Perfect Position

and the one most likely to give her an orgasm during intercourse—and it doesn't get much better than this "reverse cowgirl" position. The pluses for him: a great view of her bottom (or the treat of bobbing breasts if she faces him), the chance to relax, and (oh joy!) watch his penis disappear inside her. If she plays with herself, and flicks her hair around, life just doesn't get any better.

She wins on top because she's got control and is able to alternate between constant clitoral contact or G-spot focused thrusting. In the reverse cowgirl, she can hang on to his calves or ankles, push back, and grind against him. Most women move in a circular fashion, side to side, or simply rock back and forth, clenching their thighs and PC muscles to maximize sensation.

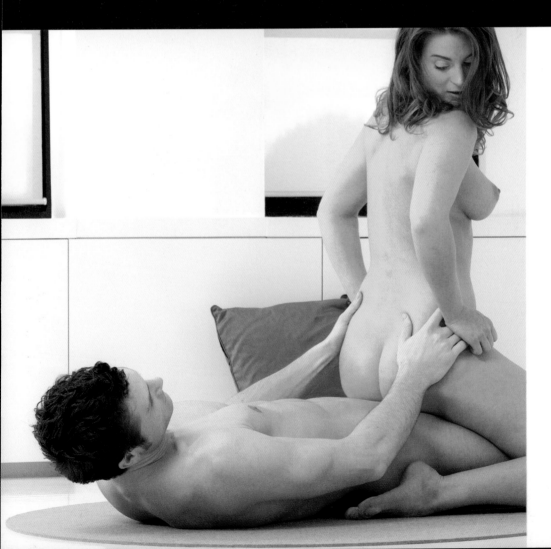

The House That Sex Built

you're having it with. (Unless it's Patrick Dempsey, then it could be anywhere, anyhow, and still be fabulous). Move the mundane missionary position to the bathroom floor and suddenly it becomes more primitive than killing a beast with your bare hands.

You've probably christened each room, what about the doorways? He leans against the doorframe, she backs on to him, pushing her bottom high in the air, going on tiptoes to allow him to penetrate. Start looking at every space, surface, and item of furniture in your house as a possible place to have sex. Improvise. Put pillows under bottoms, knees, or chests, use stairs and chairs. If you're really keen, invest in some quirky but clever purpose-built sex furniture (see pages 180–181).

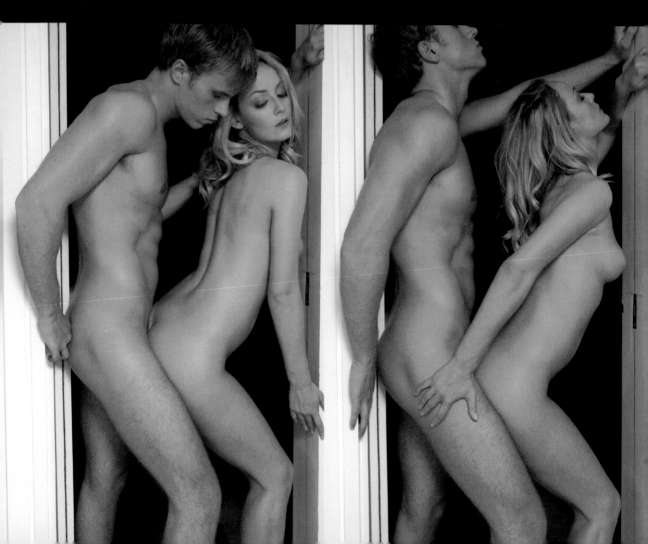

8 DIY Kama Sutra

In this scrumptiously snuggly position, she lifts one leg high so his penis hits a totally different spot. It's an example of how simple alterations can make dramatic differences. The ultimate sex position is one that feels good for both of you, depending on your height, weight, and mood. So don't just listen to me, create your own!

All positions are derivatives of the basic five—her on top, him on top, from behind, side-by-side, and standing—customize by trying different angles, thrusting styles, and pace. Remember, one person's heaven is another's hell—some women relish the show-off appeal of being on top, others hate their jiggly belly and prefer to be taken from behind, bent over pillows so it's hidden and supported. The test: does it feel like you "fit" and do you feel confident? If it or you feel awkward, forget it.

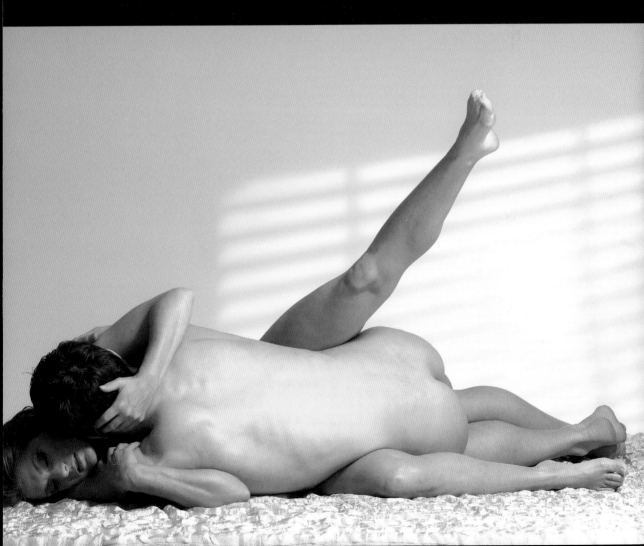

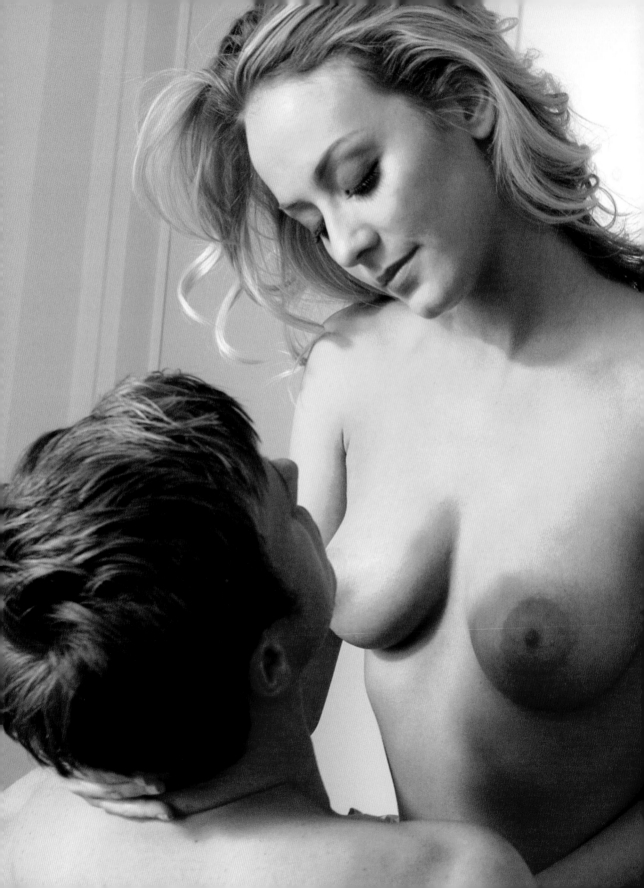

Chapter Three

Living It

17 Sinful Sex Tricks

Testicle-teasers, hand-job hints, champagne showers, and other killer combinations. Try out these signature sex moves to make you stand out from the crowd.

1 Sell yourself

Write a menu of services you're offering as a "sex worker," with a description of what each service entails and how much it will cost. Your partner gets to pay for what they require with Monopoly money.

Have a "Naughty" box in your bedroom where you put suggestions of slightly "out there" things you'd both like to do (but that you may be too shy to say out loud). Write your wishlist down, then fold the paper so there's an element of surprise when you're in the mood to take a walk on the wild(er) side.

2 Tease his testicles

Play with his testicles during oral sex or a hand-job, and squeeze them during intercourse (pull your legs up to allow yourself access). Keep the grip firm but not too tight. Try cradling them both in one hand, then circle the flat palm of the other hand over the surface. Or place your hand, palm up, under his testicles, then, with the other hand, use your thumb and index finger to make a fairly tight ring at the top of the scrotum. His testicles will then rest in your palm, neatly together. (Picture a bag of marbles with a drawstring pulled tight at the top and that's how it would look.) A slight downward tug feels exquisite and also smoothes out the crinkly skin, making them nice to stroke. Alternate the stroking with fondling and massaging.

Put both of them in your mouth together by getting him to straddle you, testicles dangling over your mouth, then circle the top with your fingers in the same "drawstring" fashion. Pull them down slightly and take both of them into your mouth, then lick and lightly suck them. You can do one at a time if you prefer, but don't be afraid to get your face nuzzled in there to do a proper job!

3 Get her to open up

If you think she's body confident and you want to up the ante during oral sex, pull back and push her legs open. Wide open. Not so wide she feels like a wishbone about to be snapped but wide enough for her to feel totally exposed. Look down at what's in front of you, ordering her not to move, then start masturbating yourself. It's very smutty. Very sexy.

Even more dramatic, get her to put her legs together, hold them straight and in the air, toes pointed toward the ceiling. Push your hands against her bottom and lift her so you can lick her vulva and anus from underneath. Then let her back down, letting your hands slide to her thighs and opening them so she ends up on her back but with legs wide, wide open and still in the air, toes pointing to the ceiling. Being "opened" like this is highly erotic because it's so "unladylike" to expose herself— you're getting a better view than she's ever had!

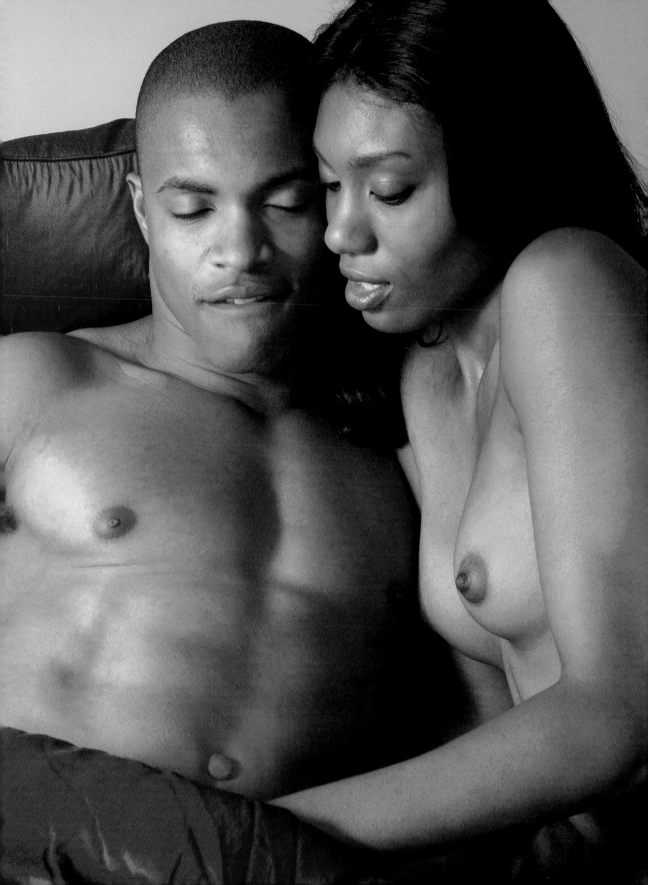

4 Champagne shower

If you're worried about the smell or taste of him (and if he's clean and healthy, stop being silly right now), give him a champagne shower. It's pretty easy to get away with this without looking too practiced, cheesy—or obvious that you're secretly washing his whatnot. Simply open a bottle of bubbly and make sure your glass is full and close by. Then take a mouthful before encasing him in your mouth. It feels great his end—the bubbles fizz and it's all terribly celebratory. You're happy because you're essentially giving him a little wash (and bet this is one time you won't complain about swallowing). The alternative to using champagne is to grab some chocolate spread and smear it over him. Why chocolate spread? It's sticky as sin and takes a while to lick off. And it's just chocolate in another form. (Though quite honestly, I wouldn't recommend the chocolate spread thing for a first time. Too distracting, and too "fun." You want the first time to be lusty and not too messy.)

5 Brave boy's oral

Add G-spot (see pages 58–63) stimulation to oral sex. Get in the traditional pose (her lying on her back, you between her legs) and insert one or two fingers inside her (while continuing to lick), upturned into a hook shape so you're aiming toward her tummy. Stay shallow—half a finger depth only—and feel for a spongy area. Press firmly (and I mean firmly for this), then make a "come here" motion. Now here's where it can get a bit tricky. Lots of women feel the urge to pee just before a G-spot orgasm and since your mouth is positioned directly over ... well, let's just say it's not a great thought for either of you. Get her to pee before the session and only try it with oral added if she's climaxed this way before.

6 Killer combo

Add anal and ball play to fellatio to give him the ultimate in head-jobs. Get him to stand while you kneel and start with oral, then press the flat of your tongue against his anus, flutter it against the opening, then make your tongue stiff and push inside, thrusting in and out. As you do this, continue stimulating his penis with your hand. Come back to his testicles by licking all the way along

Train your tongues

Do tongue push-ups to make sure your tongue is as agile as possible for oral sex. Repeat all of these exercises 10 to 20 times before moving on to the next set.

- Stand in front of a mirror and curl your tongue up so the tip of it touches the roof. Now move into a tongue curl: curl the edges of your tongue and then let it go flat.

- Next, do a tongue stretch, sticking it out as far as it will go, then pull it back in. Finally, try to touch your nose then your chin.

- While we're on the topic, cucumbers are quite handy for her to practice oral sex moves on, particularly if you're trying to master how to deep throat. (Peel it first, by the way.)

- When you're "training" each other, fingers are fabulous for him to demonstrate what fellatio tricks he'd die for her to try; her tongue can swirl, lap, or circle his palm to illustrate what would send her to sensory heaven.

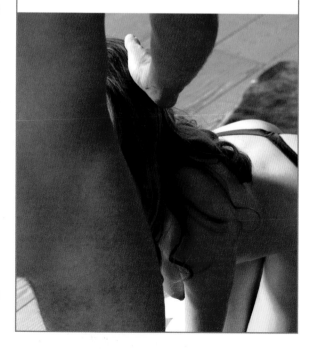

the perineum, then use a wide, flat tongue to lick them. Run your tongue up the length of his shaft and swirl your tongue around the head. Keep fellating him but add anal by inserting a well-lubed finger inside him just before orgasm. The squeamish (you or him) can get a similar effect by using the side of your hand and pressing up hard in between his legs.

7 Squeeze to please

So says my friend, Ian Kerner, one of the top US sex therapists, and author of the infamous *She Comes First* and *He Comes Next*. Every time you want to slow things down a little and prolong the pleasure, put the tip of the head of his penis in the center of your palm. Wrap the rest of your hand around the head and give it a good firm squeeze. The squeezing action pushes blood down from the tip of the penis and decreases the chances of him tipping over into ejaculatory inevitability.

8 Play chopsticks

If you've only got a large vibrator but want to intensely stimulate a small area of her (Gosh! I can't think where!), grab something long, hard, and narrow like a chopstick. Hold it loosely in one hand with the tip against the part you want to stimulate (her clitoris perhaps?), then hold the vibrator to the base of it.

9 Double the pleasure

Aim to stimulate two spots simultaneously—penis/anus, penis/testicles, vagina/clitoris, etc. It ignites twice as many nerve endings and ups anticipation of what you'll do or where you'll go next. Most of us can masturbate ourselves to orgasm more effectively than our partners (we've had more practice). The reason why it feels so much better when someone else does it isn't just because it's less effort, it's because their touch is (hopefully) unpredictable. Research shows men produce significantly higher levels of testosterone when being touched by someone else, not themselves. This perhaps explains why teenage boys try sitting on their hands before masturbating to make them numb. Easier to pretend it's someone else's hands touching it. (Hilarious.)

I wouldn't recommend the chocolate spread thing for a first time. Too distracting, and too "fun". You want the first time to be lusty and not too messy.

10 Fake a foreskin

If he's uncircumcised, he's got a built-in natural lubricant—the foreskin. Take a firm grip, then hitch a ride, gliding it along the shaft, rolling it up over the head and back down. If he's circumcised, imitate that foreskin feeling by masturbating him using a silky hair scrunchie, your (pre-worn) silk panties, a stocking, or even a slippery hanky (if you're really hard up). Wrap it around the base of his penis and roll it up and down. A strand of pearls (check there are no rough edges) also works well.

11 Don't miss out

Horny during your period but hate the mess? Soak a small sea sponge in water, squeeze out the excess, and insert it high in your vagina during your period. There's less chance of blood coming out during oral sex (though you can always insert a tampon and push the string inside) and although there's a chance he'll feel it during intercourse, it's not unpleasant. Afterward, reach in and pull it out and rinse with cold water.

12 Nicely narcissistic

Get your partner to stand in front of a full-length mirror (or catch them in the act of admiring themselves). You come in, stand behind, and seduce them in front of it. Play with their nipples, kiss their neck, run your hands over their body, remove their clothes, and yours, before pushing and rubbing yourself naked against their back. At no point are they allowed to turn around or you move

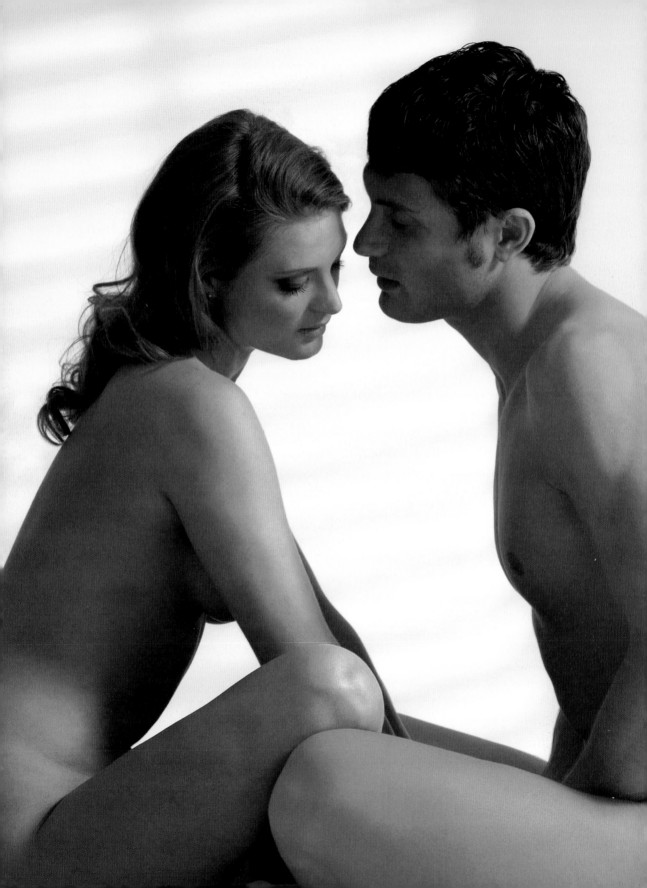

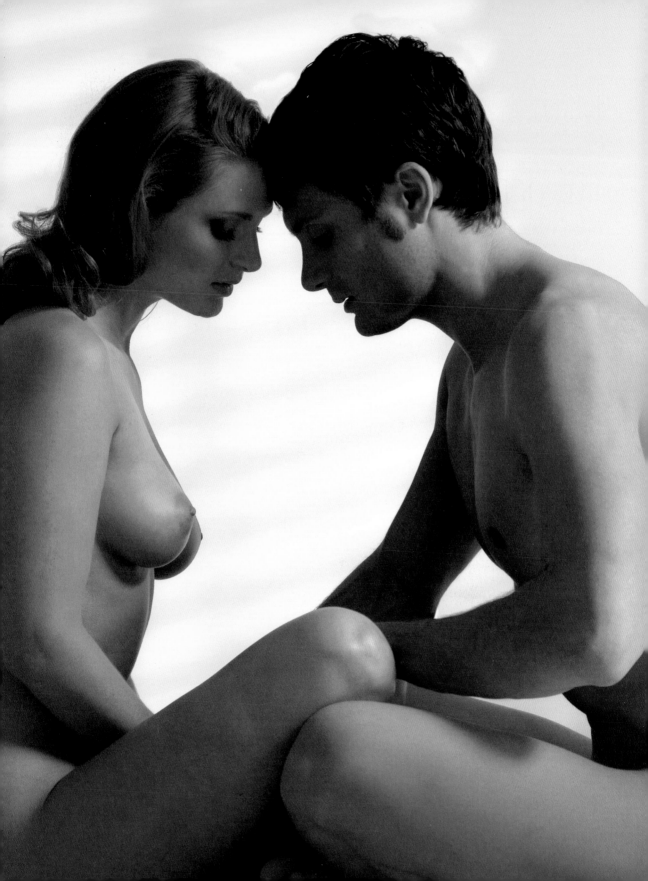

in front of them. Finally bring them to orgasm by putting your hands around them to deliver a hand-job they can watch. It mimics the angle they use when they pleasure themselves—and they get to gaze in fascination at what they look like when aroused and having an orgasm.

13 Get her wet

There's a small, sensitive area of skin at the top of the vagina close to the cervix called the anterior fornix erogenous zone (the "A" spot). Stroke this spot and she'll lubricate almost instantly. Find it by inserting one lubed finger into her vagina as far as it will comfortably go. Keep your fingers relaxed and rub gently. Use the whole length of your finger to explore the front wall of her vagina—the bit underneath her tummy. When you hit the spot, she'll start to get wet. Also try inserting your index and middle finger, then arch your thumb back, like you would if you were hitching a ride. Push your fingers inside until your thumb rests on her clitoris then thrust your fingers in and out while your thumb strokes across the clitoris. Gently twist your hand and thumb.

Make it even hotter by getting her to straddle you and then slide yourself inside but instead of her moving up and down on your penis, get her to slide back and forth. She shouldn't lift up, just rock her hips. Encourage her to start slow and speed up as she becomes more aroused (though makes sure she doesn't become so enthusiastic she's bending you uncomfortably or crushing those precious you-know-whats). It feels amazing her end and pretty good on yours as well, since it's being gripped and massaged firmly. The trick is to keep deep inside her—don't let yourself slip out.

14 Milk him

Lube up both hands (though not too much) and grab him around the base of the shaft with a firm fist. Move your hand from the base to the head, letting your hand slide off completely at the end. Before that hand's left him, however, your other hand takes its place at the bottom to repeat the action. Alternate hands so it becomes a smooth, continuous motion. Then reverse the direction so you're doing the same thing but starting at the head and moving down.

15 "V" for victorious

The "V" technique works because it stimulates parts of the clitoris that can't be seen. Use your index and middle finger to form a V sign and slide them either side of the clitoris, running them up and down over the outer labia. Your fingers should be pointed "down" (toward her bottom). As you draw your fingers up and down to stimulate her "inner" clitoris, you'll be drawing her clitoral hood lightly up and down as well, so also stimulating her "outside" clitoris. Circle your fingertips gently as you slide in the V finger position to do both at once. This technique works well during intercourse (see page 70).

16 Hot hand-jobs for her

Lube up first, then try …

- **Circling:** use the pads of your fingers to make big circles around the clitoris, making them smaller when she's aroused enough for more direct stimulation.

- **Drumming:** lightly tap along the length of the labia.

- **Stirring:** put two fingers inside her (usually the middle and index) and pretend you're stirring something. This effectively stimulates the entire vaginal wall.

- **Zig-zag:** move one or two fingers gently but rapidly from side to side across the head of the clitoris. You can manipulate the hood across the clitoris to do this if she finds it too intense. Alternatively, "march" your fingers—move them as if you're walking really quickly.

- **Pressing:** with two fingers inside her, put the heel of your other hand on her abdomen, just above her pubic bone and press down. The added pressure feels great—even better if you try it with a strong vibrator.

- **The Ultimate:** this has some less charming nick-names. "The shocker" and "Two in the goo, one in the poo," to be precise. To do it, insert two fingers (middle and index) into her vagina and another (usually the little finger) simultaneously into her anus. Your other two fingers curl out of the way. It's called "The shocker" because some men do it when their partner's not expecting it. (But you wouldn't dream of doing that, would you now?) Thing is, while some women do get massively turned-on by this, you're probably going to get better results across the board by combining clitoral stimulation with anal (insert a finger inside her anus while giving her oral), or clitoral and vaginal (fingers inside her, thumb circling the clitoris).

See page 91 for more on hand-jobs for her.

17 Hot hand-jobs for him

Again, lube up first, then let him have it:

- **Juicing:** if he's uncircumcised, hold the loose skin taut at the base of his penis with one hand, hold the shaft with the other, and slide upward. Squeeze and pulse several times on the way up.

- **Racking:** hold the base of his penis with one hand and his testicles with the other, palms turned to face his body. Now move your hands away from each other—one hand strokes up the shaft, while the other hand pulls down across his testicles.

- **Interlock:** interlock your fingers and cross your thumbs. Put his penis in the middle, then glide your hands up and down the shaft, rhythmically squeezing your hands together as you do.

- **O yes:** make the letter "O" with your thumb and index finger, place it around the corona (the ridge around the head) and twist. (Don't worry if he's too big for your fingers to meet.)

- **The Piston:** when he's fully erect and you don't mind if he orgasms, start adding in a few quick handstrokes, from bottom to top and down again, fast and hard. Then go back to whatever you were doing before. The quicker you want him to orgasm, the more you increase the number of piston strokes.

- **The Polisher:** using plenty of lube, take the base of his penis with one hand and put the open palm of your other hand on top of the head of his penis. Close the top hand around the head and twist to and fro.

See page 97 for more on hand-jobs for him.

Make him hard

This is nicknamed (aptly) the "circle of heaven".

– While he's still soft, hold the base of his shaft with one hand and place the flat, lubed-up palm of the other on the head of his penis. Letting it lie sleepy and sweetly on his belly, slide the whole thing, clockwise, so it's pointing straight down.

– Flatten your palm again and continue in a clockwise circle, moving his penis up to the starting position. You might need to swap hands to get this to work.

– Once he's aroused, switch to pinching the loose skin at the base of the penis, pulling the rest of it taut. It'll be way more sensitive to your touch.

– If he's taking a while to come, change your wrist action. Try letting it go limp or do the opposite and make it stiff—both affect the feel of the technique you're using. Also vary the pace. Go tortuously slow for a few strokes, then add in fast, hard strokes for 10 seconds before going slow again. Twist your wrist when you reach the head.

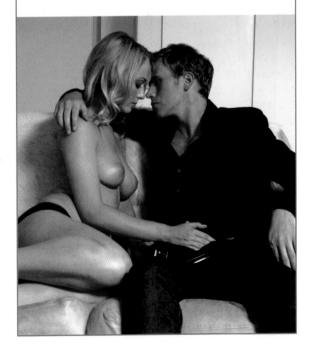

Treats for him:

Cop a quick feel

Hump his leg

Cook naked

Flash him

Push-up bra

Play solo

Stockings

Be his fantasy

Reverse strip

Sex alfresco

Try some tantric

Lollipop lick

Hot tub sex

Let him spy

Treats for her:

Suck her fingers

Cup her breasts

Play prisoner

Tie her hands

Bite her lower lip

Spank her

Take her hard

Rent a room

Tell her stories

Do it on a beach

Standing-up sex

Rent erotica

Buy a vibe

Lick her breasts

What Men Need To Know

For any man who's ever wondered what the hell to do with a naked woman, here's the truth, the whole truth, and nothing but the truth. Brace yourself, guys!

It's a lot easier for women to please men in bed than it is for men to please women. Why? Well, you're straightforward and we're complicated. And that's the understatement of the millennium. It would sometimes be easier to scale Everest than orgasm with you a lot of the time. As well as having a sexual system so complex some of its owners don't get it, women are slaves to hormone-driven libidos more unpredictable than lottery numbers. We also managed to score a huge helping of the cheery trio of self-blame, self-doubt, and self-consciousness. Add a touch of body dysmorphia and you'll get a vague idea of what it's like to be a female in bed. Bloody horrendous. Well, some of the time. Of course, with the right person, on the right day, feeling up, confident, and horny, it's a completely different story.

And this is what this feature's about—teaching you how women work, so you can make every day and every sex session that good. Well, except perhaps any that fall around day 22 or 23 (see page 91). Actually, I'd avoid even phoning then, but don't tell her I said that for God's sake. So here's what you need to know:

About her body
The clitoris is the only organ on the human body designed specifically and purely for pleasure. The head has more nerve endings per square inch than any other part of the human anatomy and two to four times more than the head of a penis. Hah! (Come on, I'm allowed a little gloat given all the above!). You can see some of the clitoris—the hood, the shaft that hides under it, and the glans (head), which is the little pea-sized tip most people think is the clitoris. But hidden from view are other bits. Imagine the clitoris as an eagle, perched at the top end of the vulva, with the shaft as the bird's body and its wings spread to straddle both sides. These wings are called clitoral legs and they're made of erectile tissue, which means they pump full of blood, just like your penis does, when she's aroused. The legs are about 2–3.5 in (5–9 cm) long and run down the sides, pointing in the direction of her bottom. But wait there's more: there are also clitoral bulbs of erectile tissue underneath the inner lips of the labia. This is all extremely good news. It means rather than one tiny area, there's lots of her you can stimulate—either directly or indirectly—to get her hot and bothered and thinking you're a great lover. Which is, let's face it, the reason why you're reading this.

About her orgasm
We talk a lot about how it's difficult for women to orgasm but the fact is, a lot of us (me included) can orgasm in five minutes or under given the right technique, lover, and/or tool (namely one that vibrates). With some skill, sensitivity, and practice, female orgasm can be easy to achieve. The reason why it's *not* that easy most of the time is because the right technique isn't to thrust your penis in and out of her vagina (which is what most men have grown up believing). The right lover is one who's prepared to use his tongue, fingers, and pelvis in very specific girl-friendly maneuvers—most men either aren't practiced in or don't even know. And the right tool is a vibrator, which a lot of you find more threatening than

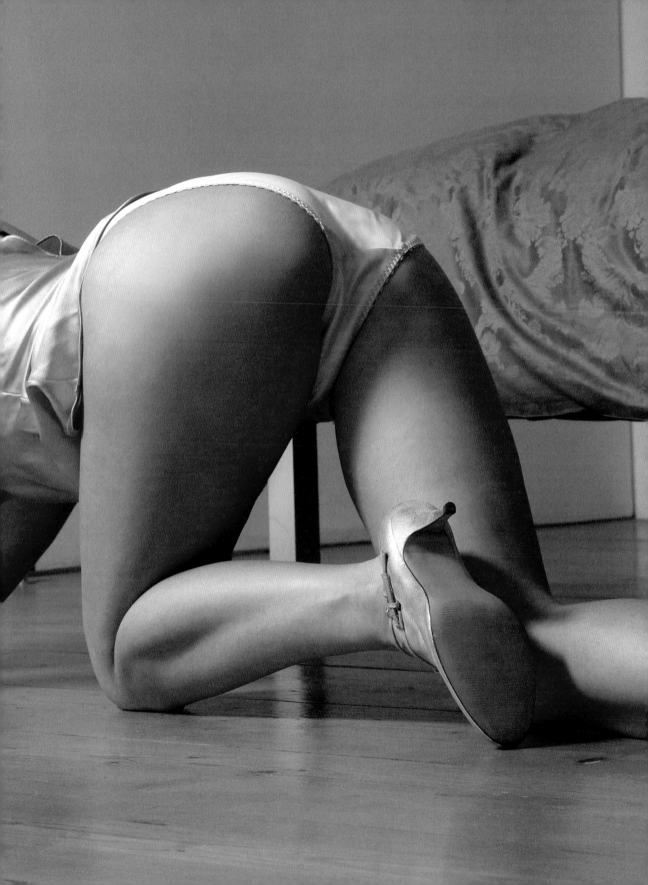

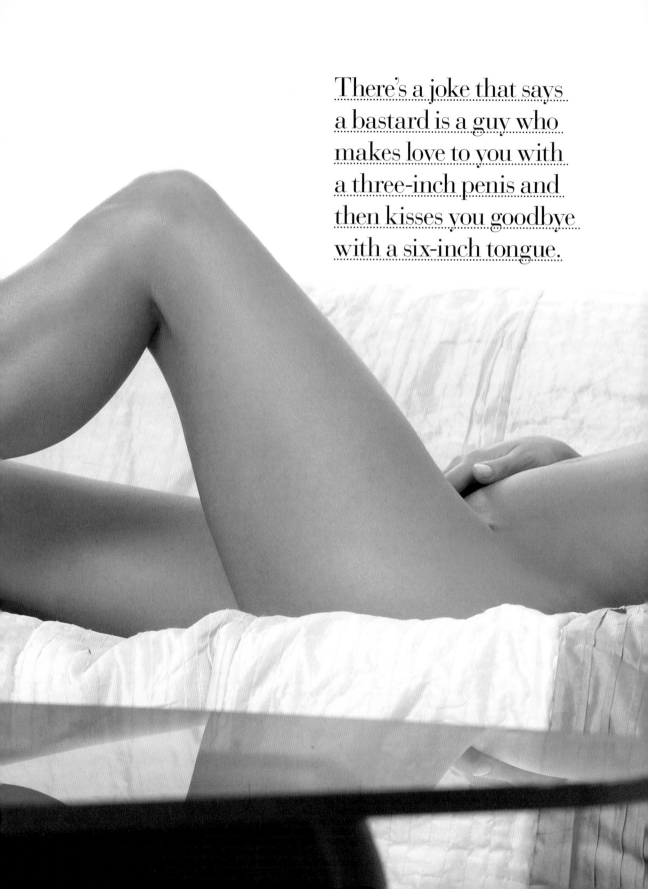

There's a joke that says
a bastard is a guy who
makes love to you with
a three-inch penis and
then kisses you goodbye
with a six-inch tongue.

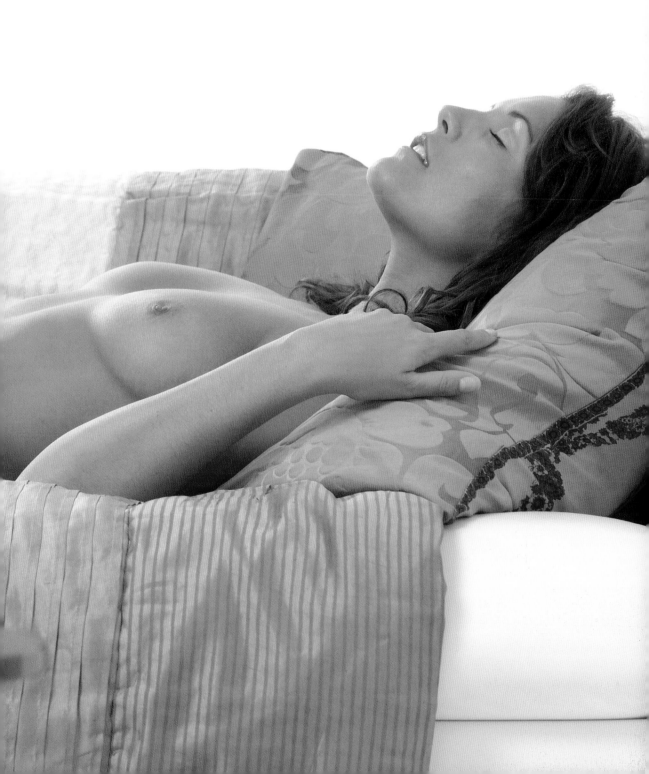

The easiest way for her to have an orgasm

Your ego's going to take a bit of a bashing here, so take a deep breath and then repeat after me "I can handle this" ...

- In a survey of more than 500 women, 34 percent said masturbating with their fingers or rubbing against something was the easiest way to climax; 14 percent said using their vibrator. That's nearly half of all female orgasms achieved without you in the country, let alone the room!

- The next most reliable method, at 14 percent, was receiving oral sex (at last, you get a look in!).

- Just 6 percent of women said they could orgasm from intercourse alone (read that again, just so it sinks in), though 12 percent managed it if there was added clitoral stimulation (fingers or a vibe).

- The much quoted statistic of it taking 20 minutes of stimulation for a woman to orgasm isn't wrong, it's just a generalization. Even sexpert Kinsey, all those years ago, knew it only took the average woman four minutes when masturbating. Your statistic has remained pretty constant—two to five minutes of direct penile stimulation to orgasm.

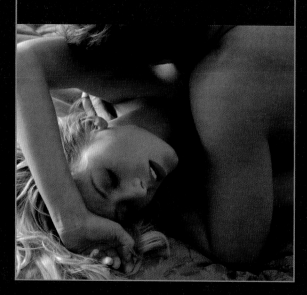

a boss hovering around your desk when you're late and hungover. In fact, you'd be more inclined to ask them to join you in bed than you would what's in her bedside drawer. As an astute male, you'll realize all of these things are solvable. The techniques on how to make her orgasm are easy to master (for tips on intercourse orgasms see page 51 and for a lick-by-lick guide to oral see pages 40–43; hints on hand-jobs are on the opposite page), but I'm talking attitude. Specifically, accepting what is going to work and what's not. Like, forget most of what you've read about all the different kinds of orgasms she can have. There is only one type of orgasm, though there are different means of reaching it: through direct clitoral stimulation of the head of the clitoris, direct or indirect stimulation of the hidden part of the clitoris (as explained earlier), or through cunning manipulation of her G-spot (see pages 58–63).

It's not a matter of a few random rubs and tugs (you lucky buggers), but practiced, focused methods that require a knowledge of how the female body works along with what does it for her *specifically*. Some of you (the ones who wear the "How do women orgasm?" T-shirts, with "Who cares" written underneath) will be putting down the book at this point, off to the bar for a beer and a moan. The rest of you may feel quite, well, hopeful. Turns out women aren't as mysterious as you thought—you really can learn how to be a good lover!

About her libido

There's a misconception about male and female sex drives. Men are supposed to get an erection putting a coin in a vending machine, women are supposed to feign a headache the second we glimpse a bulge in your jeans. Both are wrong. The main difference in our sex drives is to do with when and why we feel like sex. Because of hormones, women feel like sex lots at certain times of the month and less (or not at all) at others. Your sex drive tends to be more consistent and spontaneous. You'll feel aroused, then instigate sex. Our sex drive is more stimulative. This means we might not feel like sex at all but once we start having it, desire kicks in. This means she'll be up for shagging you senseless and doing filthy things at a particular time in her cycle (see opposite), but consider so much as a tongue in her mouth highly offensive at others. It also means it's worth giving it a try on "sort of interested" days because she might perk up after some skilfull and tactfully timed foreplay.

About hand-jobs

Let's start with some obvious basics like you've washed your hands, made sure your nails are trimmed short (universal female hatred—men with even slightly long fingernails. *Ewwwww!*), and gathered up some essentials like her vibrator (just in case) and a tube of lube.

A word on how wet she is before we go any further. Just as you can be so turned on you're pawing the ground but still don't have an erection, the same is true for her and lubrication. It's affected by so many things—cold medication, time of the month, how nervous she is, how much she's drunk—so don't assume she's not aroused if she's not sliding off the bed. Having lube handy takes the pressure off (saliva works but doesn't have much staying power). Add a good dollop and she doesn't have to worry—plus it feels *lovely*. Now, bear in mind all that you've learned so far—that it's not about penetration but about the clitoris—and you won't commit the classic guy error of thinking a hand-job is about shoving your fingers in hard and deep, because clearly what she's *really* hankering for is your penis.

The second classic error is not to ask for feedback or directions. Do this by waiting till you're a few minutes into the basic technique, then ask "Should I go harder or softer?" Wait for her answer, then ask "A bit slower or faster?" Ask "Is this OK?" rather than make it a specific question and all you'll get back is "Yes" if she's a bit shy (and you'd be surprised how many women are!). For practical techniques on what you're supposed to do with your fingers, see page 82.

About oral sex

There's a joke that says a bastard is a guy who makes love to you with a three-inch penis and then kisses you goodbye with a six-inch tongue. Whenever women are forced to choose between oral sex and intercourse in surveys, they invariably choose the tongue over the penis. See pages 40–43 to learn all of it *by heart*.

About intercourse

Note how little mention it got in this entire article! Now what does *that* tell you? Listen, I'm not saying women don't absolutely love it. Sometimes, there's nothing better than a good old-fashioned pounding (could do

When she will most feel like having sex

The following is a rough guide to what could be in the cards but for a more accurate assessment, get her to keep a diary of her erotic moods and where she is in her monthly cycle.

Days 1–11

Day one is the first day of her period. Most women aren't eager for "period sex," others are totally up for it. The week after it's over (days 6-11), forget it. Her hormones are more interested in ensuring the lining of her uterus is nicely prepped for the arrival of your semen. Remember, Mother Nature is interested in pregnancy, not pleasure!

Days 12–16

Prime hit-on-her time! This is the most fertile period for most women (be warned, some may ovulate before or after this time), which makes it the horniest. The days before and during ovulation are the days to suggest that threesome/sex on her boss's desk because the combination of high levels of oestrogen, testosterone, and lots of slippery cervical fluid combine to skyrocket her libido.

Days 17–28

Oestrogen drops after day 17 but progesterone climbs, so lots of women get a second rush of lust. Jump on her around day 20 because it's around day 22 or 23 that PMT (or what turns your lovely girlfriend into She Devil) kicks in. And you don't want to be making any unwanted advances then, do you? Her period kicks in a few days later and the whole thing starts again.

A word of warning for those of you cutting this out and taping it to the bathroom mirror. This assumes her menstrual cycle is 28 days. It's a magic average—a bit like one that says couples have sex 2.2 times a week. Having said that, it should give you a clue as to what is likely to be going on in her groin (and her head). If she's on the pill, the hormonal fluctuations aren't as noticeable, which

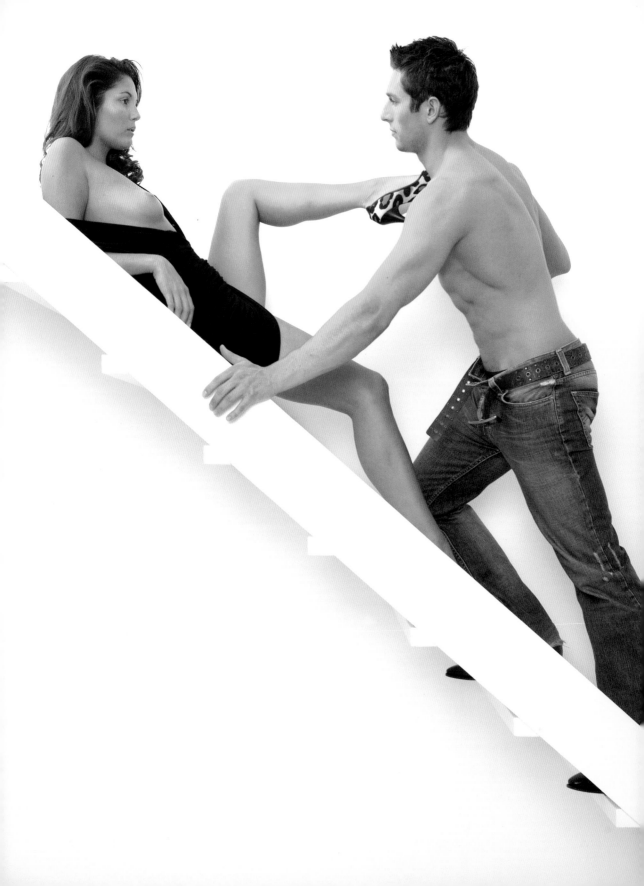

What Women Need To Know

Ready, willing, and able, right? You might be surprised. Far from being swaggering sexual studs, a lot of men want and need erotic clarity.

So there I am, in my apartment, on my fifth date with this Italian guy who had a face that was visual chocolate— you just wanted to dive on it and eat him! What I was actually hoping for was the reverse. Which is why I was (oh so innocently) putting each of his fingers in my mouth while we were snuggled up on the sofa watching a movie and (deliberately but subtly) licking and sucking them. The invitation could not have been more obvious than if I'd written "Give me oral sex now please" on my forehead. (Actually, given his struggle with English, it would have been less obvious.) So, why then, was he pretending to be completely immersed in the DVD when everyone knows the whole point of watching a DVD early on in a relationship is to provide background noise while you have wild, rampant sex. But the same man whose long, slippery tongue gave my tonsils a thorough cleaning on the first night, was *not* going there.

I found out why weeks later, via my Italian friend Luca, who'd introduced us. Once he discovered what I did for a living, he got scared. All well and good to approach women with your hands poised to polish their breasts like doorknockers when it's a pretty good bet you know more about sex than they do. Quite another thing if the woman writes books about it. "But I told him I wrote sex books!" I told Luca. But turns out he thought I said "sad books" and knowing I had a psychology degree, figured I wrote books about depression.

This did clarify why he felt compelled to explain in extraordinary detail how he was feeling each time I asked "How are you?". But what about the legendary Italian machismo? "Even Italian men are not, how you say, love-making machines," Luca sniffed in a patriotic pissed-off fashion. "You write sex books so you are scary woman and he was scared."

Pfizer, the company that make Viagra, did a survey in 2000 that found 59.2 percent of Italian men were insecure about their sexual performance, and 42.6 percent admitted to sexual difficulties. The results made headlines worldwide because Italian men are lauded for their virility, swaggering arrogance, and enormous sexual egos. Turns out, in reality, they're sexual scaredy-cats, just like the rest of us. The moral to this sad, sorry tale is this: forget any preconceptions you may have about men (Italian or otherwise) being sexual studs who are up for it with whoever, whenever, regardless of whether they've just finished a marathon, have one last dying breath, or their team's about to score. It isn't true. Men—and their penises—are vulnerable. Which means they can feel just as anxious about performing in bed as we do. And fear is not a great lust motivator. Which is why you need to get your head wrapped around his sexual insecurity before you wrap your legs around his waist.

Every time a woman asks, "Do I look fat in this?," a man looks down and wonders "Am I big enough?".

He might be able to fake an orgasm but he can't fake an erection after he's just had one.

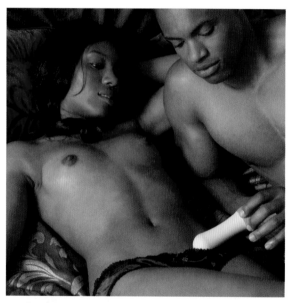

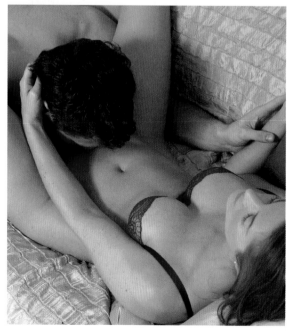

About his fears

If you have something men find intimidating—big, bouncy breasts, a face identical to an ex-girlfriend he can't quite get over, a job that earns twice what his pays, legs that seem far too beautiful to wrap around his paunchy belly—you may experience the opposite problem to what is common perception. Rather than fighting off his advances, you may have to be the one to make them. I'm not talking a one-night stand—hell, he'll be ripping that dress off the second you're in the front door. But I honestly do think sex that means something to him, that might lead to a relationship, can be more daunting for him than it is for you. Why? Well, his first worry is if his penis is big enough. It's out there remember, not coyly hidden like our parts. Then there's the worry of said penis maybe not working when he most, desperately, needs it to. Again, we can fake excitement, he can't. Or maybe it will work but too well and it's over too quickly. He might be able to fake an orgasm but he can't fake an erection after he's just had one. And all that's before he's had time to worry about what's going on with you and your bits. Say he can't find your clitoris and rubs the wrong bit and you think he's an idiot. Because it's not like he can ask for directions now is it? He's a guy! Poor bastard. This is why the next point is also critical ...

About giving him instructions

He won't want to admit it but he's depending on you to take charge a little. He wants directions and wants to give you pleasure but he doesn't want to ask for fear of looking stupid. Every man you sleep with wants to be the best you've ever had for both selfish (ego) and sweet (he really does want you to be sexually satisfied) reasons. This isn't just a male thing, we're just as guilty as men are for thinking we're somehow born great lovers. But society also casts men in the "boss" role. We know that got thrown out along with him being the sole bread-winner, but it's still hovering in the background, waiting to step forward when he feels under pressure. Now, while I'm all for giving instructions, it's a good idea to disguise them at the start when egos are at their most fragile. An easy way to do this is to deliver instructions smothered with compliments. "God, that feels fantastic," before you put your hand over his to show him how you really like it done, then "And that feels *amazing*" when he gets it right. The serious PowerPoint slide presentation complete with laser pointer can come later.

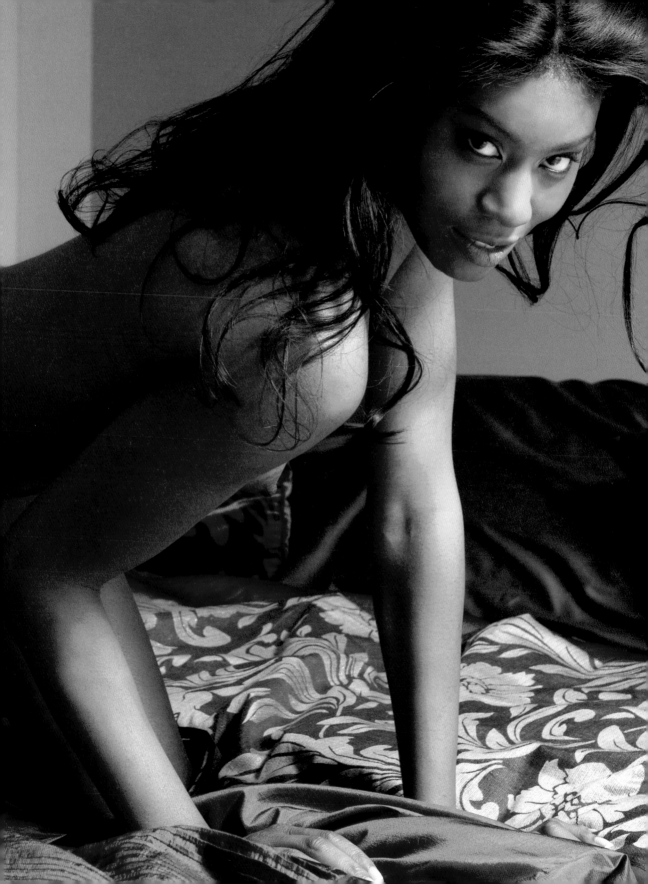

About his testicles

He might love his penis, but he's protective over his testicles. There are few things a man fears more than a knock to the crown jewels—and for good reason. Testicles are intensely sensitive and vulnerable. So is it any wonder that lots of men are a tad nervous when you head in that direction? Another reason for him to be innately defensive: they're quite important for other stuff too …

– Ninety percent of the male hormone testosterone originates in the testicles before it enters the bloodstream and travels through the body.

– The left testicle, by the way, hangs lower and is larger than the right in about 75 percent of men because the left one descends first during birth.

– They also don't sit perfectly balanced because it would be painful—damn near impossible actually—for him to walk comfortably.

– The testes hang outside the body and bob up and down toward your crotch depending on the temperature. It's hard work being a testicle— they're constantly trying to stay at the perfect temperature to produce healthy sperm!

– Every man's testicles are sensitive to pain, but sensitivity does vary individually about as much as it does in female breasts. Some men pay people to put weights on their testicles and stretch them so far, they practically hit their knees. Others run a two-minute mile in one if you so much as stroke them with a tentative finger.

– Although there are two testicles, think of them as one. Separating them by trying to pull them apart won't be appreciated. (Except, perhaps, by the guy who's paying to have weights attached.)

– He's not as obsessed with the size of his testicles as he is with his penis, but he certainly won't mind you telling him he's on the large side, if indeed he is. The expression "That took balls" means they are equated with courage.

About his obsession with size

Chances are you've figured this one out all by yourself. Every time a woman looks in the mirror and asks herself, "Do I look fat in this?", a man looks down and wonders "Am I big enough?". The "official" length of an erect penis is hotly contested (perhaps because so many of the people measuring care so much) but an accepted average is 5½ in (14 cm), with the range spanning 5–7 in (13–18 cm). A flaccid penis comes in (ahem) at around 3.7 in (9.4 cm), ranging between 2–4 in (5–10 cm). Interestingly, since width is what women see as more significant (nearly all the sensitive nerve endings are in the first inch of the vagina and a wider penis touches more of the walls), there's far less contention over this one. The diameter of a flaccid penis is around 1.25 in (3.2 cm) erect he swells to 1.6 in (4 cm). His penis is all grown up by the time he turns 17, by the way, and while you actually can't predict how big he'll be by looking at his nose, hands or feet, whipping down Dad's trousers might do the trick since heredity and genetics do appear to influence penis size.

What's also true is the "shower" (bigger than the rest of the boys when unexcited, hence the desire to show it off in the locker room) or "grower" (catches up when he is aroused and the lads are no longer around to see it— well, unless he's gay) theory. It is indeed true that you can't tell how big he might be erect by looking at him flaccid. The longest penis recorded in history was 13 in (33 cm)—and that's just the external bit. Just like the clitoris, a lot of the penis is out of view, running internally back toward the pelvic bone. This is why pressing his perineum feels great—you're massaging his inner penis. The reason why I'm arming you rather than *him* with all this information, is that you're the one left with the job of reassuring the man who feels less than adequate. Most men way overestimate the average size, few realize different sizes will fit because vaginas are elastic.

About his libido

We might all pretend it's not true but pretty much anyone over the age of 30 has figured out men are as likely to want "just a cuddle" as women are, if they're feeling stressed, tired, or vulnerable. Men are also just as likely to need bright, shiny new sex to lure them away from the television in a long-term relationship. A lot of this whole "Mars and Venus" stuff is bull. Men and women are more similar than we are different.

About hand-jobs

We all know no one can give him a better hand-job than he can himself. Which is why you absolutely *must* make him show you what technique and stroke he uses to masturbate. Pay particular attention to where he positions his hand at the start—that's the trick to replicating what he does. A common male masturbation technique is for him to form a ring with his thumb and index finger and put it around the coronal ridge—the bit where the head meets the shaft—pulling it down to the base and then back up. Other guys will wrap their whole hand around the shaft at the base and slide it up and down in a loose fist, squeezing harder toward the top and letting their thumb give a little flick as it glides. Imitate his technique as closely as possible, though that's not to say you can't try others—see page 83.

Make hand-jobs hotter

Use lube—not so much that there's no friction, but enough to keep things nice and slippery. Don't let him rush you—you set the pace rather than let him thrust and keep the strokes slow to start with. Squeeze harder than you think you should. As a general rule, what you think would hurt him feels good to him. Maintain an even rhythm but mix up the strokes a little, keeping some of them short and others long.

And always remember

The firmer and more rhythmic you are, the quicker he'll usually orgasm. As a general rule, keep your grip loose for fast strokes and tight for slower ones.

About making sex dirtier

It seems apt to end on something lots of women fail to appreciate and it's this: we spend our lives desperately trying not to be the slutty girl he can't take home to meet Mom, forgetting the slutty girl is the one he can't wait to show off to the boys at the bar. While I wouldn't suggest you turn up to your next date looking like Courtney Love on a bender, I would suggest you do this: be "nice girl" (marriage material) in public and "bad girl" (fantasy material) in private. Behave like a "wife" if you want to in front of others but do both of you a favor and act like a mistress when you're not.

– Let him see how naughty you are: masturbate for him, shave off your pubes, wear a push-up sexy bra during sex. Excite his eyes.

– Let him hear filthy stuff: play porn in the background, moan, talk dirty, tell him how much you want him when you're out (possibly whispered, rather than announced to the group).

– Let him touch you like a bad girl: in places he never dreamed you'd let him go.

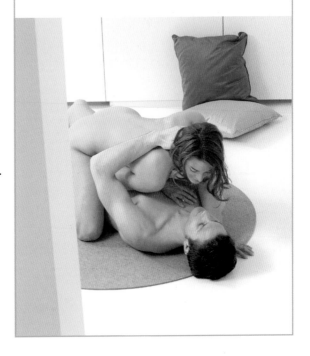

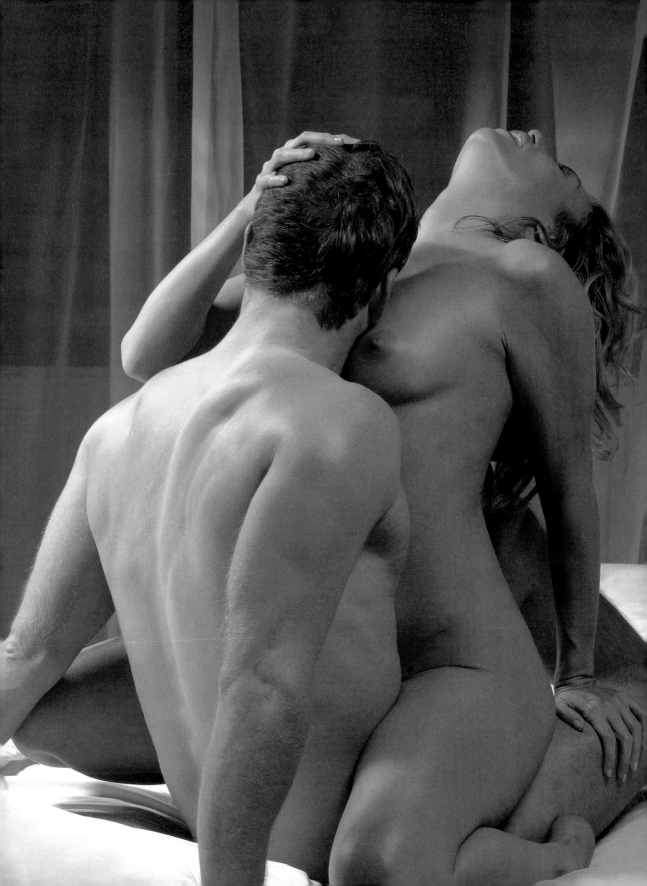

Missing In Action

Men rarely have problems reaching orgasm through intercourse—women usually do. But rethink the way you're supposed to climax as a couple and you might just get somewhere ...

Here's a question for you: What do you think is the biggest and most damaging myth about sex that's not just alive and kicking but looking like it's *never* going away? How about the fact that most women don't orgasm through intercourse and only 30 percent are able to orgasm. You've heard this before? Well, you don't have to be terribly sexually savvy to do the math once you know orgasms come via the clitoris: one clitoris *outside* the vagina plus one penis *inside* the vagina equals no orgasm for her. The reason why the myth prevails even with this knowledge is that no one truly believes it. Why would we, when women fake it so often? Why fake it in the first place? Because everyone else does and if we don't, we worry he'll think we're a freak. Women are so used to faking it, we even fake it during oral sex and manual stimulation!

Seventy-seven percent of women find it easier to reach orgasm alone rather than with a partner, even when we're including the infinitely more reliable tongue and finger techniques. Even girls who have the guts to show their partner the technique that does it for them, often cave in at the last moment because their partner doesn't do it for long enough. After demanding he does something a certain way, they say it feels wrong to also demand he does it for longer. Can you hear my groans of frustration from there? Seriously girls, when was the

last time a guy said to you, "Honey, you must be exhausted doing that for so long! I insist you stop giving me a head-job now." Studies show men actually prefer to be told what to do and don't mind doing it for a reasonable period. The reason they stop way too soon is simply because it takes much less time for him to orgasm and he assumes you're the same. Tell him it can take up to 20 minutes to reach orgasm during oral and chances are he'll relax and settle in. And you won't need to fake it. During intercourse, be very specific about what you need—his fingers, a vibrator, a certain style of thrusting—and tell him how long you need it done for. And you won't need to fake that orgasm either. If we all stop faking orgasms and sabotaging our sex lives, we might just start having one with him.

So what of the 30 percent hands-free girls—the ones who genuinely do seem to orgasm through intercourse? Some believe they're having penetration orgasms through internal stimulation of the "G-Spot" (see pages 58–63). (Lots, by the way, argue the G-spot is effectively still part of the internal clitoral structure.) Others say they're only able to do it because they're using girl-friendly pelvic grinding that tugs the clitoral hood or puts pressure directly on the clitoris. This is backed up by research. The more sexually educated, experienced, and assertive the woman is, the more control she takes and fuss she makes to get everything just right during intercourse, the more likely she is to be having real intercourse orgasms.

If she's sexually uneducated and passively lies back while he thrusts in the usual manner, those moans are more likely from frustration than frenzied passion. The more sexually insecure the woman, the more likely it is she'll fake an intercourse orgasm, believing the only reason she's not having one is because there's something wrong with her—or him.

Well, I'm here to tell you that there's nothing wrong with either of you. It's anatomy and physiology that make intercourse orgasms difficult. The very good news is this: change the way you think you're supposed to orgasm with him and you might just make it happen. This basically involves thinking of his penis and pelvis as more of a masturbatory tool—something to rub and stimulate your clitoris with and against—than an appendage that thrusts (ineffectively, if pleasantly) in and out of your vagina. Sounds selfish? Sorry to be blunt but who cares? He won't. He'll end up climaxing one way or another, believe me! And for once in your life, you might too.

But first let's first address solo orgasms. More specifically, how to have one if you never have before. Because if it's hard for women who regularly orgasm to climax in a couple, imagine what your chances will be if you've never had one at all …

How to have an orgasm

Your first orgasm is almost 100 percent likely to be achieved solo because when you've got your "learner's permit," you feel a lot less self-conscious on your own. You have complete control over what's happening and you're not worried about what your partner's thinking or how you look. I've actually never met a woman who didn't have her first orgasm solo through masturbation. It's pivotal—not just for having your first but for keeping them (and you) coming. Practice makes perfect. One of my girlfriends can take herself from a completely non-aroused state to orgasm in 20 seconds using her fingers. "I've been doing it every day since I was a kid—of course I'm good at it," she says. The more you masturbate, the easier orgasm becomes. Before we launch into the practicals, there are a few things to consider ...

– **Are you sure you haven't had one?** Yes, this is rather an odd question since your answer is probably, "Like hullo! If I had, I'd hardly be reading this would I?" But the thing is, thanks to the press and porn where orgasms are both explosive and desperately dramatic, some women imagine it to be something far more

Think of his penis and pelvis as a masturbatory tool—something to rub and stimulate your clitoris with and against.

intense than it actually is. Have you felt a buildup of pressure and any contractions at the peak of it, no matter how small those contractions? If so, you might be having orgasms, just "small" ones. You can build the intensity of your orgasms by improving the strength of your kegel muscles or building up to higher levels of arousal before letting go.

– **Are you willing to have an orgasm?** Willingness is the first stage of sexual arousal. You must want to have feelings of sexual pleasure for them to happen. If your thoughts are negative—sex is bad, I shouldn't be doing this, my body isn't good enough—it's not going to happen. The brain is a sex organ. How's your body image? Women who are anxious about their bodies tend to have lower sexual desire and enjoy sex less.

– Do you secretly think sex is dirty? Most women learn to orgasm by masturbating. If you're from a strict religious background or had parents who told you touching yourself was dirty and deviant, chances are you didn't do it. If you still find it hard to masturbate, try normalizing it by calling it (and sex) by another name. Using a word your brain doesn't instantly associate with "bad" makes it less threatening. Try calling sex "having fun" and masturbating "giving myself a present."

– **Educate yourself about your body.** One of the best and clearest diagrams of the female anatomy is in The Elusive Orgasm by Vivienne Cass (which is handy since the rest of the book will be rather useful to you as well!). Armed with the book or another good diagram, take a mirror, have a good look at your genitals, and find your clitoris. You'll also need to go online (or brave the sex shop) and buy a simple but powerful vibrator (the non-penetrative type—see pages 138–143) and some good quality lubricant (available at any pharmacy).

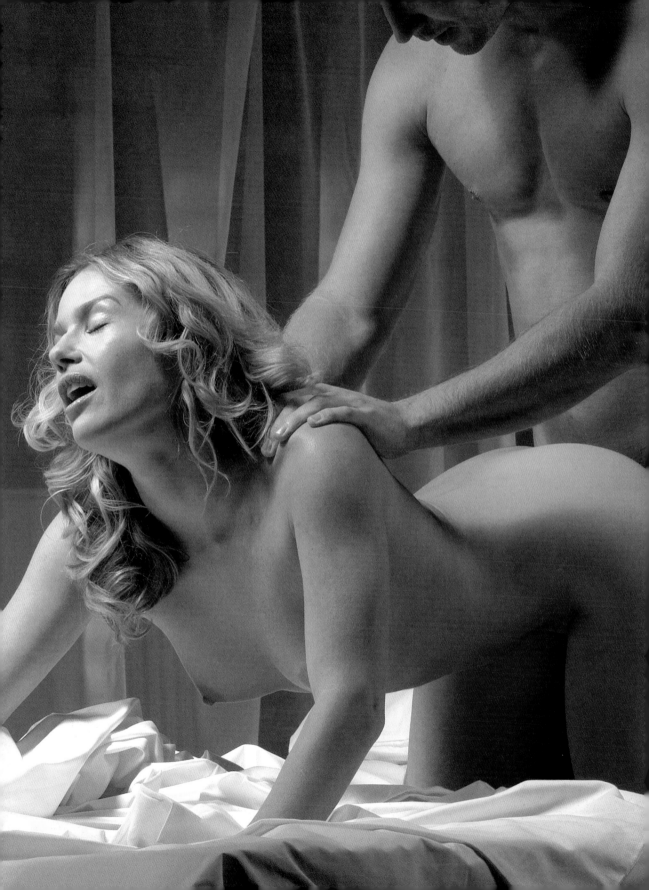

When was the last time a guy said, "Honey, you must be exhausted doing that for so long! I insist you stop giving me a head-job now."

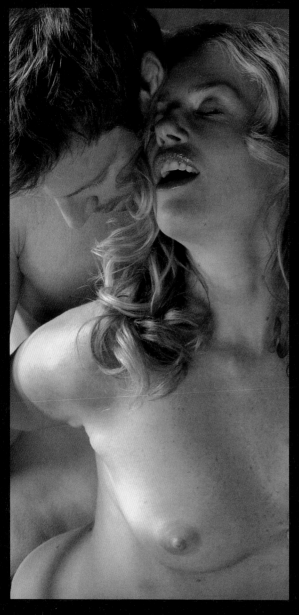

– **Have a vibrator orgasm** so you know what you're aiming for. Some therapists will advise you not to do this and to try with your fingers first as they are partner friendly. I agree it's crucial you are able to orgasm using your fingers but a vibrator is indisputably the easiest way to get there the first time. It's pretty impossible not to orgasm using a vibrator. Hold it against the closed labia (lips of the vagina) at the top end so you're vibrating the clitoris underneath. Try rolling it, holding it at different angles, and varying the speed and pressure. It's really as simple as holding it where it feels good—and keeping it there.

– **Fight the urge to stop when pressure builds.** The feeling of orgasm is frightening the first time you experience it. I was scared—I seriously thought I was going to explode and that I'd peed myself. But all that's happening is lots of blood is pumping to your genital and clitoral area. An orgasm is simply the euphoric moment when your body releases the blood back into the body. Once you understand what's happening, you'll (hopefully) feel less freaked out by the sensation.

– **Can't orgasm even with a vibrator?** The vibrator might not be strong enough, it might be too strong (try putting a T-shirt between you and it), or there may be deep, psychological factors at play. Sometimes, an early traumatic experience you don't remember can still influence you. Our brain will "hide" information from us if it thinks it's too painful to recall. Sounds clever and it is to a point but your brain isn't the only thing that remembers: your body does too. If you feel there's something wrong but you're not sure what or feel generally uncomfortable about sex, see a therapist. A good sex therapist will usually cure any problems quickly and efficiently. Only a tiny percentage of women never orgasm once they've had professional help—you're unlikely to be one of them.

– **Say bye-bye vibrator and hello fingers.** Once you've had an orgasm using a vibrator and know what you're aiming for, it's banished to the bedside drawer. Now let's try to orgasm using your fingers. Put some lubricant on your inner lips or your fingers and first find your clitoris—the pea-sized bit, hidden under a protective hood, at the top of your vagina. Try gently stroking near or around it with your middle finger or the pads of a couple of fingers. Try moving around it in circles then gently rubbing directly across it, back and forth, once you feel more aroused. Experiment with different strokes—hard, soft, fast—until you find what suits you. Try to get to the point where you're really excited before either giving up or giving in (and letting those fingers slide over to the bedside drawer where your vibrator lives). It takes longer with your fingers until you've got the technique mastered, so be patient.

– **Keep trying with your fingers.** Aim for about six or more 15-minute sessions over the next two weeks. If it's not working, try alternative ways to masturbate: a new position (try lying on your tummy or sitting in a chair rather than lying or sitting on the bed with your legs apart), or rub your clitoris against something (like the arm of a sofa). Focus on enjoying any sexual feelings you are experiencing rather than fiercely concentrating and thinking, "I must have an orgasm." The harder you try, the further away it will seem.

– **Add erotica.** Fantasize about something you've done that turned you on or would like to do. Read a book on sexual fantasies or explore erotica or female-friendly porn (see page 157). Try squeezing your pelvic floor muscles and remember to breathe deeply. One last word of encouragement: the first solo orgasm may take ages to work up to, but it gets easier and faster the more often you have one. Promise!

Orgasm during intercourse

Here it is in one sentence: act like a man. In the brilliant book *I Love Female Orgasm*, author Dorian Solot points out what is blatantly obvious but ignored. That guys don't lie back waiting for their partners to give them an orgasm during intercourse, they do whatever it takes to get them there. They'll thrust in a certain way, rhythm, angle, or speed, do it in their favorite position, make sure they have the right fantasies playing in their heads and are looking at what they want to see. "Guys make it clear that they expect to have lots of sexual pleasure, and an orgasm, and they assume the sexual interlude will continue until they do," Dorian says.

It's up to you to do the same. Think about what you need. What position, technique, pressure, and pace, what head-space you need to be in, any "extras"

Reasons why you can't orgasm
– Too busy.
– Don't like to be out of control.
– Don't understand your body.
– Sexually inexperienced.
– Sexually unconfident.
– Unable to say what you need.
– Lack of sexual communication.
– Guilt, stress, and anger.
– A history of traumatic sex or abuse.
– Use of some medications.
– Feeling rushed by a partner.
– A bad lover.
– Painful sex.
– Bored with sex and partner.
– Don't fancy partner.

Make these changes so you can
– Make sex a priority.
– Deal with stress and upset.
– Tell your partner what you need.
– Focus on what you're feeling during sex and like about your body.
– See a therapist about sexual trauma.
– Learn to let go.
– Challenge any negative messages.
– Be selfish sexually sometimes.
– Leave a dead-end relationship.
– Get a physical check-up.
– Be healthy and energized.

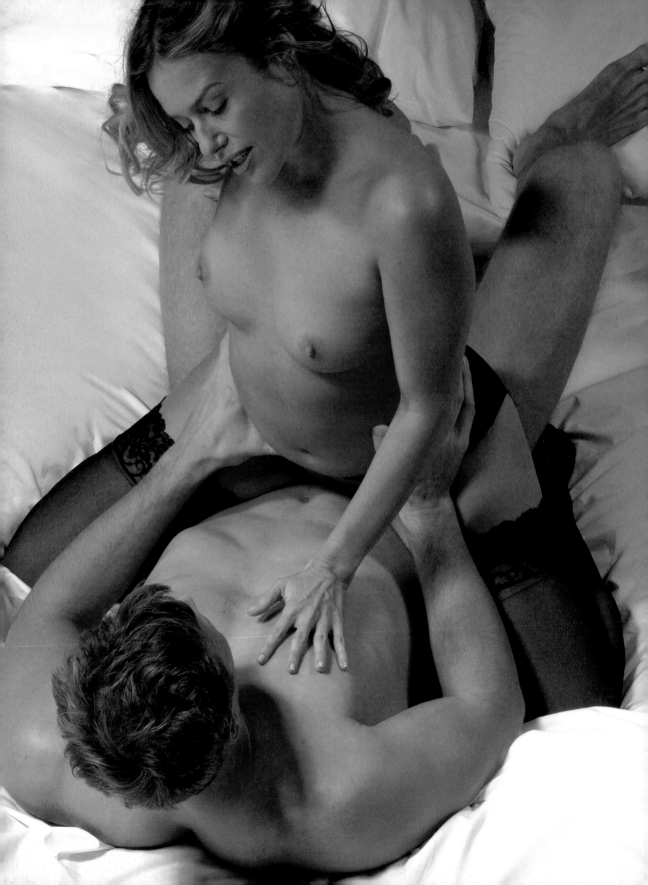

stimulation elsewhere) you need, then go for it! Be proactive. Jump on top, pull out your vibrator, put his fingers there, hump him. Think "How do I put pressure on the clitoris" and do whatever it takes to do that.

– **Have "femoral" intercourse.** Use his penis as a masturbatory tool. This works best if you're on top. Put lube on the shaft and wrap your labial lips around him, sliding up and down the shaft, letting it rub against your clitoris. A him-on-top version: you keep your legs squeezed tightly shut and he runs his pre-lubed penis between your legs and vaginal lips, grazing the clitoris. There's no penetration at all in these techniques.

– **Penetrate in stages and use single thrusts.** In *He Comes Next*, sex therapist Ian Kerner suggests this highly effective technique. The idea is to use single controlled thrusts that allow deep penetration and stimulation of the G-spot and combine it with rubbing against him for the all-important clitoral pressure. You jump on top, put just the head of his penis inside you, stop for a few seconds, then in one smooth motion, slide to the bottom of the shaft, staying there for 10 seconds while you grind yourself against his pelvic bone while he's deep inside you. Slowly pull up again, squeezing your kegel muscles around the shaft as you do. Again, stop when it's just the head of his penis inside you, wait a few seconds and then slide back down and repeat. The trick is to do this really slowly, focusing on squeezing and maintaining control. Go too fast or let him take over and he will orgasm.

– **Hold his bottom.** When he's on top, grab his buttocks and pull him close to you, massaging the cheeks so his pelvis grinds into yours providing clitoral pressure.

Jump on top, pull out your vibrator, put his fingers there, hump part of his body. Think "How do I put pressure on the clitoris?" and do whatever it takes.

On-the-edge techniques

You've got much more chance of climaxing with him inside you, if you make sure you're highly aroused before he penetrates. Try one of four techniques that are all based on this principle.

– Get him to penetrate *immediately* after an orgasm he's given you with his hands or mouth. This can set off another wave of contractions. You may orgasm more easily the second time around.

– Get him to use his fingers on your clitoris (using lots of lube) and bring you almost to the point of orgasm. He then penetrates and continues using his fingers on you, with only a few seconds break.

– After he penetrates, move immediately into a girl-friendly thrusting style. If you're intent on sticking with traditional thrusting, get him to aim for your G-spot and then cross your fingers!

– Either hold a small finger vibe or classic vibe on your clitoris while he's penetrated, get him to wear a vibrating penis ring, or consider a vibe that stays on during intercourse (see page 139).

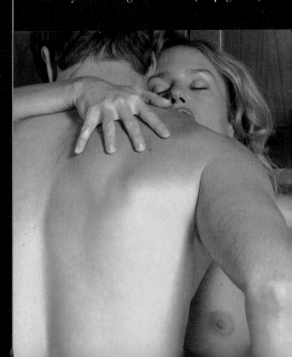

How To Have Lust That Lasts

The fairy tale says we meet, fall in love, and live happily ever after. It certainly doesn't include being so bored in bed that it's more fun masturbating than having sex with your partner. Can lust last the distance? It's not designed to … but there are ways to trick the system.

If you had to choose between being absolutely and totally in love and having a deeply satisfying, pretty sensational sex life, what would you settle for? It's a choice no one thinks they'll ever have to make—and sure as hell never wants put in front of them—but, I have to be honest, all the recent research (rather depressingly) tends to point this way. Don't jump off the cliff just yet—there are things you can do to circumvent this—but the first step does seem to be accepting that love and lust aren't quite the chummy bedfellows we thought they were. In fact, they're more like bitter enemies.

Here's why: when we fall in love with someone, we "merge" with the other person. This makes us feel all safe and snuggly and at peace with the world and our partner. Eroticism requires "separateness." What is desire if it's not unfulfilled anticipation? Desire surges to its most powerful, wondrous peak when we first meet and want someone, simply because we're unsure if our feelings are reciprocated. Once it turns out they're just as besotted as we are (be still our beating heart!), the distance that was between us disappears (be still our

beating groin—not quite so fab) and all the uncertainty, edginess, anxiety, and jealousy that kept us in that feverish, longing state is suddenly removed. Novelty, risk, and separation all up the desire factor. We want quite the opposite when we're in love so actively seek out exactly what will destroy it.

Even worse, we can't even blame each other for this because it's not the fault of either sex. As Esther Perel, author of the ground-breaking book *Mating in Captivity*, points out, "Any ideas that cast women as longing for love, essentially faithful, and domestically inclined, and men as biologically non-monogamous and fearful of intimacy should have been dispelled a long time ago. Social and economic changes circumvented traditional gender lines a long time ago." Having said that, just to make life even more difficult, each sex does bring its own particular foible to the table.

If you hear the words "Let's make love" come out of your mouth, wash it out with soap. Better still, fill it with wine and get so roaringly drunk, you scream "For God's sake, shag me!" at the top of your lungs.

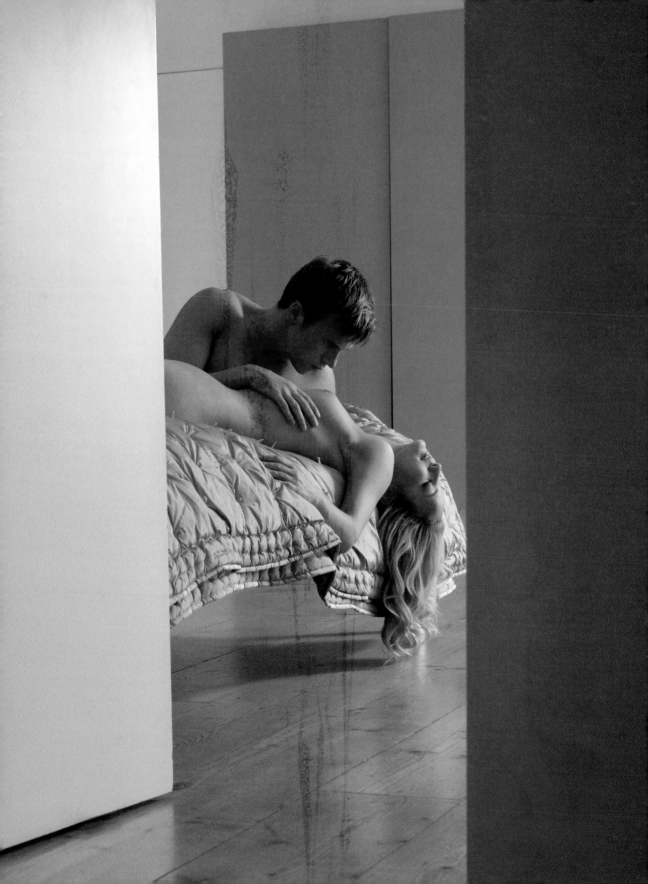

Synching sex drives

Some of us are thrillseekers, needing and actively looking for novelty and adventure. Others like familiarity and routine. You don't have to be a relationship expert to figure out this is going to cause problems. While one of you checks out "Camel treks across the Sahara" vacations, the other gazes wistfully at pictures of the sweet little cabin by the lake. Sexually, it's the same deal.

One wants to give the swingers' bar a whirl, the other would rather a nice, long bath (solo) followed by formulaic sex they know and trust. Forget what you've heard about opposites attracting; in bed it's far better to have similar sexual personalities. The trouble is, it's hard to get a true reading early on. Newness and the emotionally bonkers act of falling in love boosts the sex drive of low libido people and makes routine-loving lovers more daring. Meanwhile, the sensation-seeker is happy with "ordinary" sex because it's fresh flesh and they're high on love hormones. It's only when the hormones wear off, that you get a true picture of your natural "resting" sex drives. Can you synch sex drives for better sex? Yes, see page 113.

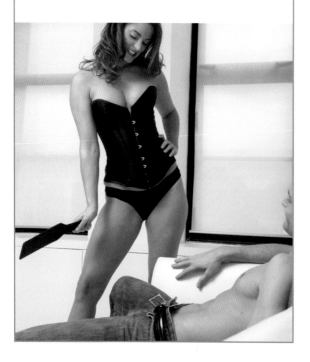

Men can't multi-task

Men are lousy at lusting and loving simultaneously for partly biological reasons. The male brain releases high levels of vasopressin when deeply in love, which, in turn, decreases testosterone, the hormone responsible for sex drive (see page 27). But loving her also means worrying about her well-being. The pursuit of pleasure requires us to be selfish little brats: become too absorbed with your partner's pleasure and you'll lose desire for them. When this happens, men often think they've fallen out of love but quite the opposite has happened. They love her so much, the act of caring is too heavy a burden of responsibility. Desire and lust makes you want to do filthy, sometimes quite degrading things to your partner. If she's sitting on a pedestal of love and respect, the two don't sit easily together. "Sex without sin is like an egg without salt," said the famous director Luis Buñuel. Take away the ability to sin and you take away desire.

Women think too much

Her desire follows another, equally disastrous, path. Female desire is often linked to how we think he feels about us. In the beginning when he wanted to slam us up against the fridge and forget about dinner, we'd be like "Fabulous! He must *really* want me. That cellulite-reducing cream did do the job! How hot am I!" Six months on, he'll do the same thing and instead of our eyes becoming hooded with lust, they'll narrow with suspicion. Instead of thinking "Great!," we're liable to think "Why?". Is he having sex with *us*, or having sex because he just feels like sex? Who's he thinking of when he's doing it? Is it leftover lust from checking out that new girl in the office?

Then the "sex is dirty" thing starts to kick in. Like, he can't possibly be thinking about us as a potential mother of his children if he's suggesting doing *that*! And that's without even touching on the how we feel about our body thing. Sigh. It wouldn't occur to men to think "Jesus! The old beer gut's looking a little large today. Better not shag the ol' lady." But, for her, one unflattering reflection in the mirror on the way to the bedroom and it's like someone put a pin in the desire balloon.

Other lust hijackers

Feeling unattractive. Hormones. Emotional history. Insecurity. Not liking your partner much. Genetics. These are just a few of the things that transpire to rob us of lust. Our baseline personality also plays a part, as does life experience. Sexual desire is a lust for life as well as sex. If you're boring or the rest of your life is boring and uninspiring, why would you leap into bed with energy and enthusiasm, a wicked gleam in your eye, and a cache of sex toys clutched in your hands? You need to be excited by life to be excited by your partner.

Love without lust

All relationships (well, possibly not one-night stands) move through three stages: lust/infatuation, romantic love, and attachment. The third stage is designed to be calmer, to provide us with a sense of stability so we can mate and procreate. (Which, let's face it, is sort of the point even if we like to forget it is.) It's around this stage that what you never thought was going to happen to you does: you're—dear God!—*bored!* So bored in fact, masturbating is more fun than having sex with your partner. At least then you can watch some porn or play out that fantasy about seducing the next-door neighbor. Suddenly, you find yourself in love but not in lust and that leaves you, well, *confused.* This isn't right! This isn't what happens in the movies! Panicked, we either cheat, leave, or settle for what we think is our lot: sexual despondency. The fact is, we're built to fall in love but not to stay that way. Only 3 percent of mammals are monogamous, the rest have serial sex or a lifetime of one-night stands.

If you're boring or your life is boring and uninspiring, why would you leap into bed with a wicked gleam in your eye and a cache of sex toys clutched in your hands? You need to be excited by life to be excited by your partner.

Why the honeymoon has to end

In "the honeymoon period"—the very beginning—everything, including sex, is pretty much perfect. But there's a reason why we don't stay bathed in those delicious infatuation chemicals (see page 26): it's emotionally and physically impossible to sustain long-term. "It's the body's innate wisdom to turn down the volume because it cannot maintain the lust-crazed state forever or people would eventually collapse with exhaustion," says world-famous neurologist and brain-imaging expert Daniel Amen, somewhat shrewdly.

– Infatuation can last anything from six months to two years but despite wearing us out, when it does make its inevitable exit, few of us are happy to say a fond farewell.

– Lots of people assume once the intensity and euphoria drops off, it's a sign they're not in love anymore. Not true. It's just your brain changing gears so it can release the "cuddle chemicals," which is when "true" love really begins.

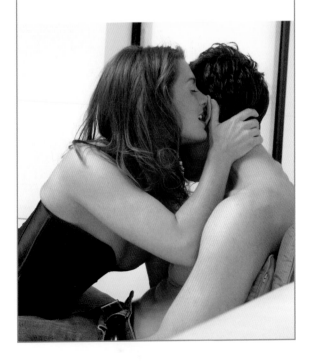

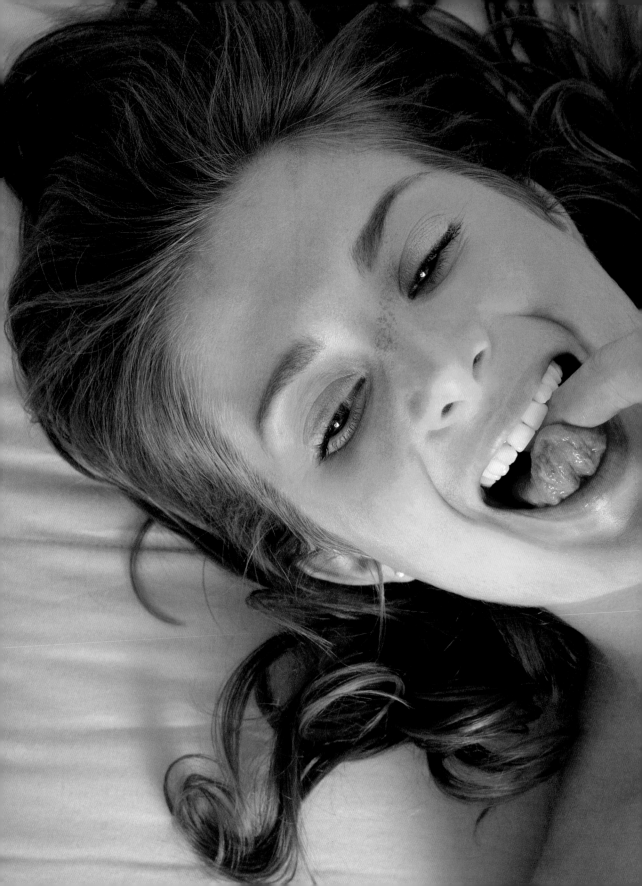

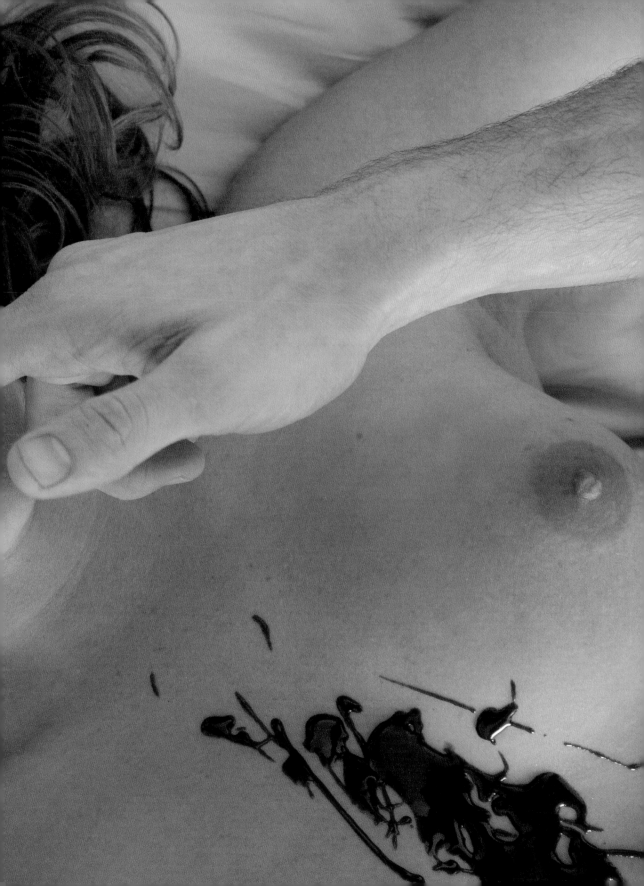

Tricking Mother Nature

For those of you who are still reading and not swinging from the rafters, the thing to realize is I'm not really telling you anything you don't already know. I'm simply explaining why. We all know nearly half of all marriages end in divorce, this just gives a little insight as to why this might be. And if we know why, we can usually fix it. Knowledge is power. It might be common but it's not inevitable that your relationship will follow this rather dire passion pattern. Here—and throughout the whole of this book—you will find practical ways to fight back. For instance, the following are the solutions thrown up by the most recent research on the topic:

- **Stop trying to live up to** society's notion of the ideal sex life and instead focus on what turns you and your partner on and experiment with that.

- **Look and act shaggable** and drop the "You should love me no matter what" attitude. They probably still *do* love you when you're sprawled on the floor in front of the TV, cutting your toenails with one hand and exploring one nostril with the other. Whether they'll suddenly get hard or wet is another thing.

- **Fantasize and stop stressing about it.** Physically having sex with your partner and mentally having it with someone completely different isn't wrong, it's what's going to stop you from straying.

- **Stop being sex robots.** When you've been in a relationship with someone a long time, you develop a "sexual shorthand." You know exactly what to do to get them off and they do you. Because it works and it's easy, you then so rarely stray from that path, your bodies know how to do it all by themselves. Effective, yes. When you're both tired or time deprived, appreciated. Exciting long-term, hell no.

- **Change location**. It's one of the quickest ways to make sex more exciting. The most familiar touch in the world feels wanton and wicked when a hand sneaks under the tablecloth in a restaurant to snake its way up our thighs. A mild petting session spirals to sizzling hot if it's done in the back of a cab. Ditto the position you've done countless times when it's on the hood of your car in the garage.

- **Trade-offs don't always work.** Promising to do it your partner's way one time, and yours another can work but it may leave you feeling resentful when it's not your turn. You may also find you get a lackluster, lukewarm response from your partner when it's your turn. The best solution is to compromise sometimes but try to find middle ground or at least blend taking turns into the same sex session.

- **Don't fall for the clichés.** Lose the idea that sex when you're single is raunchy and rampant and sex when you're married is loving and affectionate. If either of you ever hear the words "Let's make love" come out of your mouth, go and wash it out with soap immediately. Better still, fill it with gallons of wine and get so roaringly drunk, you scream "For God's sake, shag me!" at the top of your lungs. Don't feel guilty if you want to get nasty.

- **Lose the idea that it's disrespectful** to do or suggest doing filthy things to your long-term partner. Granted, there's an art to suggesting it without offending but don't let that put you off (instead turn to pages 146–153 for a few hints). So many people let go and indulge in wonderfully naughty sex with strangers but stay prudish and proper with their partners.

- **Perfect your sexual techniques** and work out physically what you each need but remember desire starts in the brain. It's as important to connect before and after sex as it is during it.

It wouldn't occur to men to think "Jesus! The old beer gut's looking a little large today. Better not shag the ol' lady." For her, one unflattering reflection is enough to put a pin in the desire balloon.

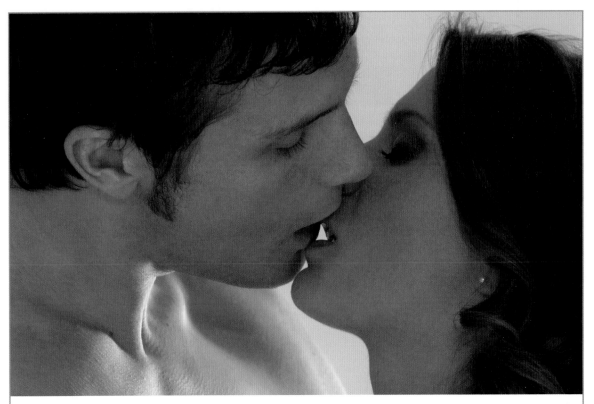

10 libido types

Knowing what intrinsically drives us sexually is vital to achieving long-term satisfaction. In *When Your Sex Drives Don't Match*, Dr. Sandra Pertot identifies 10 types of libido. Try identifying your own and your partner's libido and using it as a springboard to sorting out the kind of sex you both need to keep you interested long-term.

- **Sensual:** sex is an expression of love. Emotional intimacy is the most important thing.

- **Erotic:** sex needs to be intense and lusty. Low-key "ordinary" sex is OK but it needs to be punctuated with some extraordinary sessions.

- **Dependent:** sex is used as stress release and you become agitated if denied it.

- **Reactive:** sex is about giving not receiving. It can be based around a low sex drive or you need to see your partner aroused to become aroused yourself.

- **Entitled:** you have little understanding of your partner's sexual needs—-just believe you're "owed" a certain amount and type of sex.

- **Addictive:** sex is something you find so appealing, it's hard to manage. It controls you rather than the other way around and you're prone to cheat.

- **Stressed:** sex is worrying. You feel under pressure to perform and worry you're inadequate.

- **Disinterested:** sex provides little pleasure and you rarely desire it. It can be the result of distressing sex that's quelled any natural desire.

- **Detached:** sex is good but competing distractions put you off and you emotionally withdraw from your partner and sex.

- **Compulsive:** sex is only satisfying if you follow a specific ritual. Fetishists fall into this type of libido. It's selfish sex that involves little connection with your partner.

- **Don't be scared to add outside stimulation.** If porn's not your thing (you sure? See pages 154–161), written erotica might be. Dip into a classic D.H. Lawrence or try Nancy Friday or Black Lace books—reading out bits from a sexy book can be excruciatingly erotic—especially for women, since research suggests we're more turned on by words than visuals. Others you might like: *The Naughty Bits* by Jack Murnighan, for the steamiest, scandalous sex scenes from the world's best books. Or *Full Frontal Fiction*, a collection of short, sassy, modern stories. While we're on the topic, don't dismiss good old-fashioned dirty magazines. They're portable porn (easy to access and hide quickly) and a good way to introduce a shy partner to watching adult films. There are as many specialized magazines as there are individual sexual tastes.

If you've stopped having regular sex

- **If your relationship has changed** from lovers to friends, make a pact to become sex partners again. Rule out any health or emotional problems that might be interfering: medication (anti-depressants?), anger in the relationship, painful intercourse, erection issues. If you need to seek professional help, do it. Did you both just fall into complacency or did something happen to stop you regularly having sex?

- **Decide on obvious "I'm up for it" signals.** If you're a touchy, feely couple and also ultra-considerate (she's tired, bless her. I'll just massage her shoulders and see if it leads to anything), it's easy to miss each other's tentative little sexual overtures. Work out some that are so obvious that even the cat knows what's on the agenda for the evening.

- **Start sending those signals.** You have to have sex to want sex. One of the best ways to break out of a sex rut is to just close your eyes and go for it even if you seriously, seriously couldn't think of anything worse. Act on a mere flicker of desire.

- **Get over the idea** that you're both somehow going to be instantly aroused just by looking at each other. That happens at the very, very start when it's all as romantic

as a Disney movie (with very rude bits thrown in). It's not going to happen when you've already done it to the same person and body 20,000 times. Pounce on every opportunity—most particularly his morning erection. While we're on the topic of erections, you both also need to give up on the idea that he's going to get an instant erection every time he so much as thinks about sex. Again, that's how things worked at the start—like when you were 18—not 28 and over. Lots of men need to be physically stimulated before an erection appears, it may not just happen automatically.

- **Introduce some quickies.** I know I'm like a stuck record on this one but I swear to God if you make yourselves have sex three times a week for five minutes each time, it will kick-start your libido.

- **Consider getting professional help.** Wait for desire to kick in. If you haven't had sex for a while, doing it again will feel weird. But you should start to feel some type of connection after about a month if you're seriously trying a few new things, talking honestly about it, and doing it on a regular basis. If after all this, you're both still nonplussed, you might like to consider seeing a sex therapist. It sounds drastic, but what can take months or even years for the two of you to figure out, could be sorted by them in a couple of sessions. Find a good one and you'll be making whoopee like you never dreamed possible in no time at all.

The most familiar touch in the world feels wanton and wicked when a hand sneaks under the tablecloth in a restaurant to snake its way up our thighs. A mild petting session spirals to sizzling hot if it's done in the back of a cab.

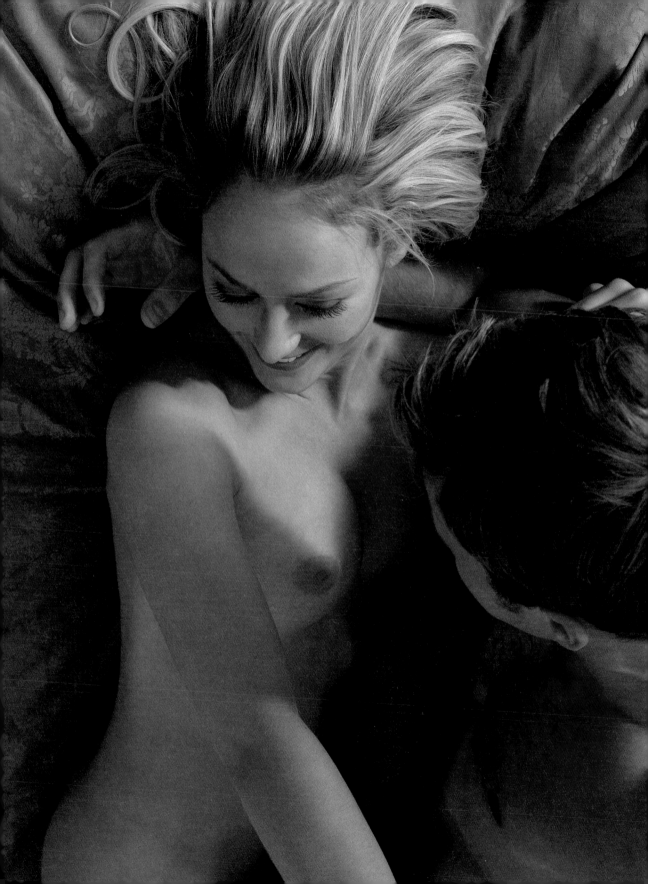

Instant Sex Make-Overs

Want to fix your sex life—now?
Transform your love life tonight
with these fast, easy fixes for
common couple sex complaints.

1 We Don't Try Anything New in Bed

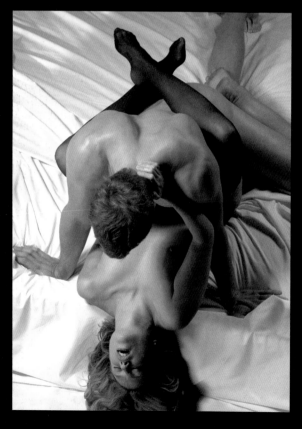

The "new" thing doesn't have to be something ultra-kinky to work. The trick is to try one or two *small* things and then build from there.

– **Go through this book for inspiration** and individually mark things you like the look of. The pages both of you have marked, you try first. The rest are negotiable once you've broken out of your comfort zones. It's not cheating to steal stuff out of a sex book rather than think it up yourself—that's what they're for! You get on with doing the dishes and let me think up what to do with those hands when you're finished.

– **Take turns to plan a sex night.** The person whose turn it is decides what you're doing—when, where, how, organizes any props, and is the instigator. This forces each of you to adopt different roles as giver and taker.

– **Add some new positions.** If you're in a rut, you're probably using one or two positions on a regular basis. Choose at least six others (see pages 64–73), and you should end up with an extra two or three that you like. Add in some of the oral sex techniques on pages 38–47 over the next few sessions, then dip into the "17 Sinful Sex Tricks" on pages 76–85.

2
I Want To Suggest A Three-Some

When it comes to suggesting a threesome, it depends a lot on the combination you want and when you're asking. Generally, the more committed your partner and the longer you've been with them, the more offended they might be. It's a natural instinct to not want to share (see page 165), which is why, if you're really into threesomes and want them as part of your regular sex life, you need to establish your partner's views quite early on. It's easy to find out: simply talk about a friend who's really into them and see how they react. They'll either screw up their noses and go "Ewwww. I so don't get threesomes" … or look intrigued.

– **Never, ever launch straight in** with "How about we have a threesome?" I know tons of guys who've made half-hearted, drunken requests and ended up losing their girlfriend or spending the next 10 years paying for it. People either love the idea of a threesome or hate it with a passion usually reserved for pedophiles.

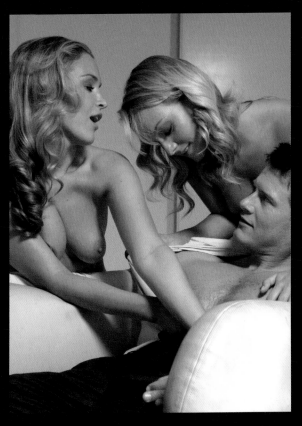

– **Even if they react favorably** to threesomes as a concept, don't be surprised if they still get horribly offended at you suggesting one. Lots of people think threesomes are fine for couples who aren't in love so, if you suggest one, your partner may doubt that you "truly" love them. Play it very much from the "I'm just intrigued by it and wondered what you thought" angle rather than "I've already lined her/him up and they're coming over tomorrow night."

– **If I had to generalize horribly,** I'd say both women and men are more open to a two-women, one-man threesome than other combinations. (Unless you're gay of course, which throws up a whole other set of combos.) Lots of women are highly suspicious of men who want her and another guy—gaydars bleeping all over the place—plus the whole "How can you share me?" thing seems worse when it's a guy.

– **What if your partner wants one and you don't?**
Try not to have the knee-jerk reaction of thinking they're bored with you sexually. It doesn't necessarily mean that, though it does mean they want hotter sex. By all means say no (in my opinion, most committed couples should—see pages 164–165) but, as a compromise, suggest going to a lap-dance or strip club and have a full-on flirt while your partner watches, or consider having phone sex with a sex worker on loudspeaker.

3

I Want Him to Use a Vibrator On Me

Some men are both sexually experienced and cool enough to accept a vibrator's going to do it for you more regularly than any part of him will. But this also assumes you've been honest about your orgasms. If he's used to giving you extra clitoral stimulation with his fingers, or knows you only orgasm during oral sex, he's unlikely to gasp with astonishment if you suggest using a vibrator during penetration. If, however, you fake it regularly and never admit to so much as masturbating, he's going to be a little perplexed as to why your twosome has suddenly turned into a threesome.

So the absolute first step is to make sure you've come clean. So to speak. The second is to make sure you own a non-threatening vibrator (see pages 138–139 for suggestions) that's not bigger than he is. Then …

– **Pull it out from under the covers** seductively and say "I know you like to watch." Use it on yourself, put on a show (and take your time—he doesn't need to know immediately that it takes you a second to orgasm with it and half an hour with him.)

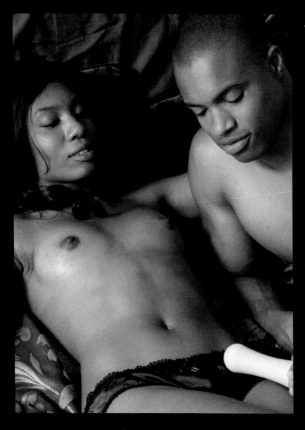

– **Once he's got used to** having the three of you in bed together, he'll be more open to using it during sex together. Bring it out a few sessions later and say "What about you?" Even if he laughingly fobs you off, just play around a bit. Buzz around his nipples. Have a laugh. To be honest, I've never met a man yet who's been hugely keen on vibrators used on his penis. Try running it on a very low speed up and over the shaft but don't be surprised if he says "Don't know what you girls are so excited about!" and pushes it away. You'll be more successful holding it against his perineum while using your hand on him—or during oral sex. Many men have turned from cold to convert by you holding it to the side of your cheek as you fellate him.

– **Once everyone's made friends,** the next step (a few more sessions on) is to wait till he's using his hand to stimulate your clitoris during intercourse, then say "Wait, I've got an idea." Then pull out your vibe. Say, "I know your poor hand gets tired." If you've been pretending to orgasm up to now say, "I wonder what a *vibrator* orgasm would feel like while you're inside me compared to the usual orgasm you give me." (Yes it's another fib but you blew the "let's be honest" thing by faking in the first place.)

4
They Hate My New Trick

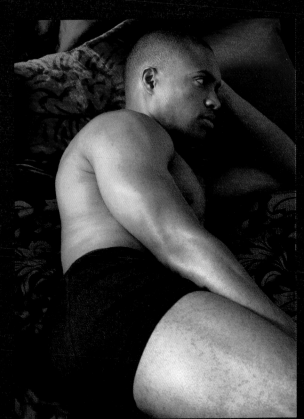

Everyone has a unique erotic blueprint, so what works for one person isn't going to work for all. Having said that, I know from experience that it's totally gutting if your signature sex move leaves someone cold. But resist getting huffy. It's not personal, it's just their personal taste.

If your partner discreetly lets you know whatever you're doing is not for them, just stop and then continue as though nothing's happened. If they react obviously or forcibly (which can happen with unwanted anal play or testicle fondling), pretending nothing's happening is a bit like denying you're having an affair when you've been caught *in flagrante delicto*.

Acknowledge it by saying, "Sorry! I thought you might like it but it's fine that you don't." If you're sensing they don't like it but are too polite to say so, stop, laugh, and say, "This isn't impressing you, is it?" If it's the other way around and you're on the receiving end, be polite but be direct—especially if it hurts or you really don't want them to go there. Simply remove their hand (penis, vibe, carrot, horse's head) and say, "Thanks for trying but I don't really like that." If you can follow it up with a positive "But I loved it when you did that," even better.

What's hot
Facing problems together rather than burying your heads in the sand. Talking things through before they get too serious. Working as a team, instead of blaming each other.

What's not
Expecting your partner to just know what you need or want and getting sulky or angry when they can't magically read your mind.

5
He Wants To Come In My Mouth

You could just agree to it! Semen's just protein and sugar—it's harmless (and no, it won't make you put on weight.) Having said that, don't let him come in your mouth unless he's been tested for HIV and STIs—all it takes is a little cut in your mouth and you're infected. If it's the taste that puts you off, it's probably his diet. The healthier the diet, the better he'll taste. (Pineapple juice is supposed to make him taste sweet, though the old wives' tale isn't terribly specific about when and how much he's supposed to drink.)

– **If you do decide to swallow**, when you feel him about to orgasm, position his penis so it's way back in your mouth. It's easier to swallow in one gulp and you'll bypass the top of your tongue, where your taste buds are. Or aim it toward the inside of your cheek and swallow quickly. If you actually like swallowing (and it's not *that* rare, by the way!), try holding his pelvis in both hands when he's near orgasm and rock him toward you so he goes deep into your mouth as he ejaculates.

– **Another technique is to pretend to swallow** by keeping your mouth or lips lightly over the tip of his penis and pressing your tongue gently against the slit at the top as he ejaculates. Continue to milk his penis with your hand and simply let the semen drip out of your mouth and down the shaft. It feels nice for him because it's super-slippery and is a good compromise: he's sort of come in your mouth but you haven't had to swallow.

– **The other option is to say,** "I want you to come *all* over me." And mean it. Let him let loose on your breasts, your face, your neck, in your hair. (Possibly time it for after lunch at his parents, rather than before.) As he's doing it, say "God, that's a turn-on."

– **The infamous pearl necklace** involves you putting lube on your breasts, pushing them together, and slipping his penis in between. He thrusts—if you can reach, lick his penis as it pops out the top (this works or soooo doesn't, depending on the size of your breasts and his penis). When he ejaculates the semen ends up around your neck, just like a pearl necklace. Except not a terribly permanent or expensive one.

– **The least exciting option** is to remove your mouth, while keeping on working him with your hand. But you're not going to choose that one, are you? Good.

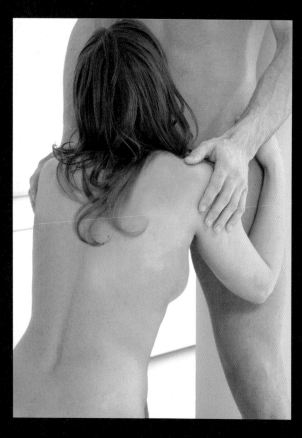

6 I Want To Have A Rewarding 69er

The concept of receiving and giving pleasure at the same time sounds ridiculously inspired but the sad truth is the fantasy nearly always exceeds the reality of a 69er. It involves *major* multi-tasking and a certain degree of unselfishness—which is why one person tends to get the better end of the deal. Literally. If they do their job well, the other person gets so lost in it, they tend to forget they're supposed to reciprocate, drifting off into a heavenly licky-la-la land until an indignant shove of the hips makes it impossible to ignore what's staring them in the face.

Men tend to like 69ers more than women—probably because they're more comfy with their bits, less squeamish about having bottoms so close to their nose, and don't have to concentrate as hard to orgasm. Make your next one more satisfying for both of you by:

– **Taking turns.** Try one of you using their mouth, the other using their hands. (Don't panic, by the way, if his erection goes up and down.)

– **For her:** if you're on top straddling his chest, him holding your hips, try rounding your back, so it's easier for him to reach you. Or put pillows underneath his head. When he's on top, wrap your palms around his penis to help control how fast and deep he goes.

– **For him:** try it side by side, your head pointing toward her feet and get her to bend her top leg back so her knee is in the air and her foot flat on the bed. This creates a triangle with her legs and means you can rest your head on her bottom thigh while you lick her.

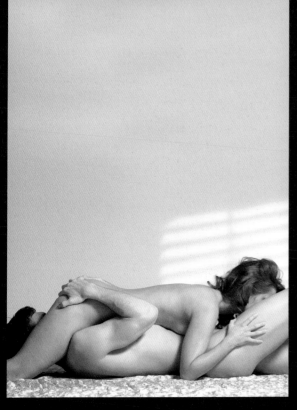

They drift off into a heavenly licky-la-la land until an indignant shove of the hips makes it impossible to ignore what's staring them in the face.

7

He Prefers Porn To Sex With Me

He's more interested in watching porn than he is jumping into bed with you? First up …

- **Accept it's not you.** Don't get me wrong, if you've dramatically changed appearance or been a total bitch, it might be you. But if it's simply happening as the relationship ages, it's probably because he's lazy. It's not necessarily because he doesn't fancy you anymore.

- **Accept you need to feed his desire.** If you've been together longer than eight months (let alone 18), the chemicals that fuel desire are already trickling to a halt. Sad but true. The good news is you can trick your bodies back to producing them. See page 112 or try out any of the tricks in this book designed to give your sex life a jolt. (That'll be the whole book then.)

- **Confront him—but in a light-hearted way.** Joke that his computer gets to see him more than you and that you bet he can't go without watching his porn for a week. Or two. He'll protest that it's easy (no one likes to admit addiction), then all you have to do is hold him to it. If it's not that bad, get him to agree to no porn on evenings when you want a little somethin'.

- **Make it obvious when you do feel like sex.** Say, "I want sex with you—tonight." One of the reasons he likes porn is that it's upfront and "dirty" so be dirty, talk dirty, masturbate in front of him. He wants porn, give him porn. Stop asking for sex, start appealing to his visual side by showing him. Walk around naked. Strip for him. "Accidentally" leave your heels on as you walk around in your underwear.

- **Don't ban it.** Ban it and you make it even more appealing than it is already.

- **Make it quick.** One reason he enjoys porn is because it's quick sex. Warm yourself up—masturbate almost to orgasm by reading a sexy book, watching a movie, or using your vibrator. Then get on top—he gets to be lazy as well as score the visual treat he's used to.

- **Snuggle up afterward.** The difference between having solo porn sex and couple sex is the skin-to-skin contact and intimacy. He might pretend not to enjoy the cuddle at the end but, in fact, he's likely to be just as enthusiastic as you are (if sleepier).

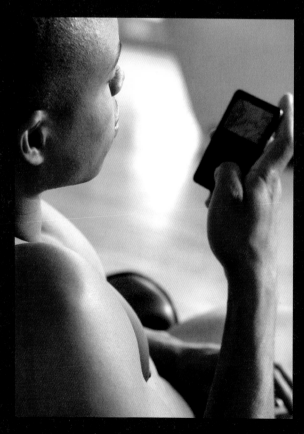

8
I Want To Last Longer

She's as hot as hell, it's the first time, you haven't had sex in ages, it's a new relationship—there are plenty of reasons why you orgasm too fast but, interestingly, no "official" time period that will define you as suffering from PE (premature ejaculation). The most-cited definition is if you orgasm too fast for you or your partner's satisfaction. To reassure you just a little, (given most of you believe the average intercourse session is 15-30 minutes), lots of men ejaculate within two minutes of penetration. Yup. That quickly. If you want to beat that:

– **Look at your masturbation habits.** Masturbation can be the friend or enemy of PE. Do it just before a sex session and you'll last longer second time around. Focus too much on the head (the most sensitive area) and you'll orgasm in record time, training your penis to rapid ejaculate. Astute when you're staying at Aunt Betty's during summer vacation, not so clever when you're shagging Britney ten years later.

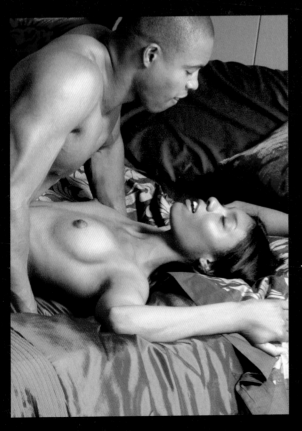

– **Control your arousal level.** Pinpoint your personal point of no return using the "peaking" technique. You learn to recognize how sexually aroused you are—on a scale of 1 (not aroused) to 10 (orgasm)—and discover what number on the scale you need to hover by to retain control. You might feel in control till you reach level 6, but know once you're a 7 or 8 it's moving dangerously close to ejaculation (once seminal fluid begins pooling at base of penis, nothing can stop you coming). Practice peaking during masturbation. Start by paying attention and trying to chart where you are at what point. In later sessions (allow 15-20 minutes per session) stop at different levels and try to control your arousal. Peaking is a new improved version of the old "stop-start" technique that simply taught you to stop all stimulation the minute you felt yourself get out of control. Peaking just asks you to be more specific.

– **Give it a squeeze.** An oldie but still a goodie is the squeeze technique (which you can use in place of or along with peaking). You (or your partner) places a thumb on the frenulum and wraps two or three fingers tightly around the head of the penis. Then you or they squeeze tightly and hold for a few seconds or until the urge to orgasm subsides. It also works if you squeeze the base firmly. Tugging the testicles downward can also delay ejaculation, as can pressing three fingers firmly into the center of the perineum.

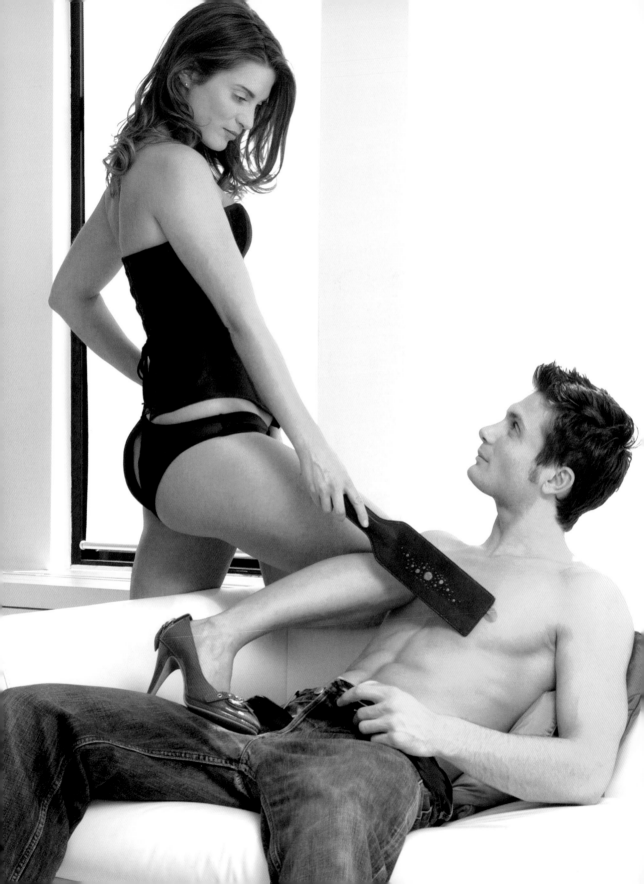

Chapter Four

Pushing It

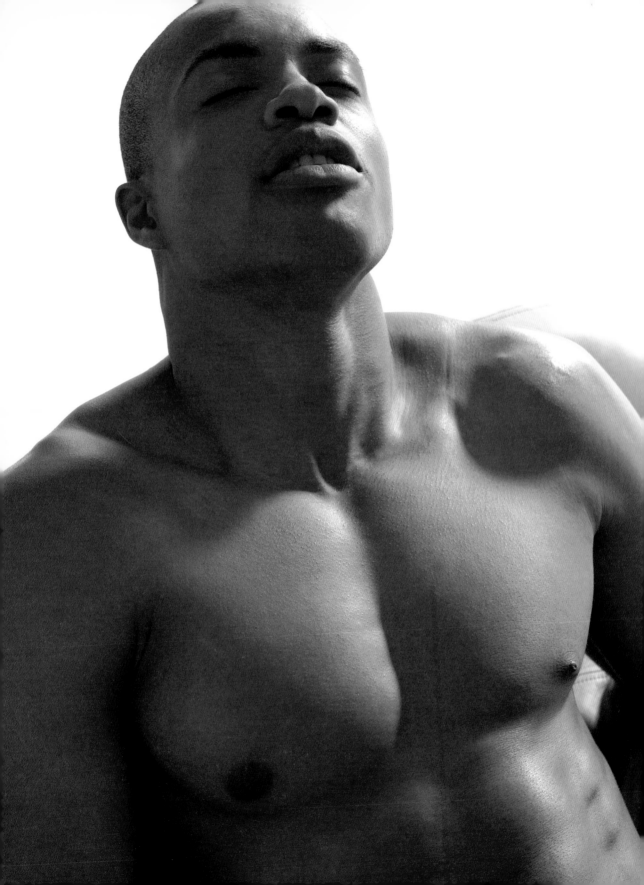

Have Sex Like A Gay Man

For years, men have been told to have sex like women. The real truth is, women should be having sex like men. More specifically, gay men …

I went to an art exhibition in London recently, which traced sex and its representation in art through the ages. Part of the exhibition included a series of photographs of various couples that aimed to capture the essence of their relationship and sex life. They were both graphic and private: intensely tender moments mixed up with them having (rather rude in some instances) sex. The first series was based on a straight couple, the second two gay guys. What struck me immediately was the difference in the sex lives. The gay guys didn't just have more sex than the straight couple, they had an extraordinary variety of it.

Different positions, locations, props. Tender sex, wild sex, using their hands, penises, tongues. They beat the straight couple's sex hands down. Why? Because it's two men, that's why. One half of the couple doesn't suffer from the female hang-up of "I can't do that, it's too perverted/unladylike/slutty." Because they think alike, gay guys know their partner won't judge them—and neither partner sees anything wrong in what they're doing!

The male sex drive is more base, primitive, and "dirtier" than a female's, so when you put two males together you get some pretty raunchy stuff. The lesson to be learned as a straight girl: the only thing standing in the way of you having great sex is your attitude! In society, there's a clear line drawn between "normal" and "naughty": what's accepted and what's not. The definition appears to be this: if everyone does it, no matter what "it" is, it's "normal" and OK to admit to. If only a few do it, no matter what "it" is, it becomes "sick" or "weird." Nonsense! Take a leaf out of the gay guy's book and refuse to live by such archaic, Victorian rules! The next time your partner suggests doing something unusual, don't have a knee-jerk reaction. Ask yourself, "What's my objection? Is it because it's just something I don't think other people do?" If it is, then ask yourself "Will this hurt us physically or emotionally? Is there any danger?" If the answer to those questions is no, then what's the problem? Be one of the few women to embrace this concept and you'll be the best lover he's ever had and is EVER likely to have.

So this one's for you girls. I am generalizing horribly in places. Not all straight women behave in the way I describe and not all gay men have great sex. I'm buying into lots of stereotypes (and as one of my gay friends said, "I'm sick of people assuming I like shopping and cocktails when I like football and beer") and for that I apologize.

Put his middle finger in your mouth. Swirl your tongue around it, suck it—do everything you'd do if it was his penis. Bar using your hand—that would be odd!

The gay way

So girls, there are lessons to be learned from gay guys and these are ...

- **Look good.** Straight women tend to dress up when they go out but relax the rules at home. Gay guys make sure they always look good. Because they take sex very seriously and want to ensure they get lots of it, gay guys pay a lot of attention to their appearance. They're acutely aware a man's desire is strongly driven by visuals—hence why gay men have the best bodies and show them off. I'm not suggesting you sit there watching *Law & Order reruns* in your LBD and high heels, but if you pull on your big pants, tie your hair back, and veg out on the couch *every night*, he's not going to be looking at you thinking, *"Umm. I might have me some of that!"*

- **He's got nipples too!** Gay guys know nipples can be a hot zone. Be warned, though, while some men love their nipples tweaked, pulled, or even bitten just before they orgasm, others hate it. Experiment but don't be offended if he pushes your hand away.

- **Give good finger.** Gay guys know finger sucking is incredibly hot! Do it in public but do it discreetly (he's facing outward, you're facing the wall). Take his hand and put his middle finger in your mouth. Swirl your tongue around it, suck it gently but firmly, move your mouth up and down—do everything you'd do if it *was* his penis (bar the fist thing with your hand—that would just be plain odd!). Maintain eye contact.

- **Jump on him.** Straight women wait till they're in bed to initiate sex. Gay guys have a more urgent sex drive. Do they care if it's the tub, bed, or kitchen sink that's used as a prop? Sex in bed is boring. Comfy, yes, but exciting, no. If you must have sex in bed, at least lure him in there at an interesting time—like when his parents are downstairs and you fancy a quickie.

- **Straight shooters.** Gay men swallow. If they decide not to, it's not because they don't like it but because they like the thrill of watching their partner ejaculate. Watching semen spurt out is more fun to them than shoe-shopping for us. Let him give you a pearl necklace (and no we're not talking Tiffany).

How to use a butt plug

It's not just male bottoms that are packed with super-sensitive nerve endings. Yours is too! Want to see what all the fuss is about? A good way to tell if you'd like to try anal intercourse is to experiment with a butt plug. See page 142 for how to choose one, then follow this simple guide. It works for either of you, but I'll assume he's doing it to you for this exercise.

- Once you're aroused (or post-orgasm when you're relaxed), get him to apply lube (see page 130) to you or the vibe (or both) and run it around the rim of the anus. Get him to gently press and see if your anus "pulls" the toy in. If it doesn't, he should press gently until the toy is inserted a little way. Even if it is "pulled" in, get him to penetrate with it slowly, stopping to let you get accustomed to something inside you. Once it's inserted—they don't go terribly deep—you just simply leave it there and continue having sex as usual.

- If you enjoy the sensation, you might like to give anal intercourse a try. In a survey of women who did, 25 percent rated it as "very pleasurable" and 38 percent "somewhat pleasurable." The rest weren't too impressed. It depends on whether it's done properly (if it's not, it hurts) and on how big he is. Some women can actually orgasm through anal sex (though it's rare), a few more are able to if there's clitoral stimulation at the same time.

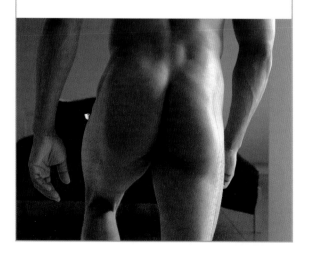

– **Encore, encore!** Straight women are often too embarrassed to let their man watch them masturbate. Gay guys like showing off—and watching other guys turn themselves on. They also watch carefully to see what technique they use, so they can copy it later.

– **Be every woman.** Gay guys are more likely to have open or semi-open relationships. I'm not suggesting for a moment that you do the same (or encourage your partner to) but it doesn't hurt to give him the illusion he's sleeping with lots of women. Do this by varying the style of lovemaking. Switch between playing an innocent, a wanton hussy, a bossy dominatrix. Adjust your underwear as well as your attitude: white virginal lace for "virgin," saucy red or hot pink for sex siren.

– **More than a penis.** If he comes too soon, gay guys don't bat an eyelid. The whole object of having sex is to get off—if that happens quickly, great! It doesn't mean their mouths or hands have stopped working— and there's always second-time-around.

– **Bedroom bores.** Straight women are too polite to say "Hurry up!" if he's taking ages. Gay guys get bored and say so. They'll try everything they can to make it happen but, if it goes on too long, they suggest he DIY while they watch. You do the same and when you do, watch to see if his masturbation technique is incredibly hard, fast, or rough. If it is, that's what's causing the problem. Get him to train himself to orgasm with you by getting himself used to a gentler grip.

– **Try a love tap.** Straight women are rarely the ones to instigate spanking. Gay guys like giving "love taps." Try doing it during intercourse—start with a light, playful slap and see how it goes down (checking he doesn't).

– **Play with power**. Gay men understand the erotic appeal of power. Look and learn. Play both submissive and dominant by tying him up and letting him return the favor. Use your stockings or try PVC bondage tape. It comes in big rolls like masking tape so your Mom can pick it up and not have a clue what it's for!

– **Stop people-pleasing.** Straight women gush about how good the sex was afterward, even if it wasn't. Gay guys don't say much at all. "Why do you need to? It's obvious whether the sex was good or terrible," says a gay friend of mine. If you feel the urge to say something, keep it simple. "You were amazing" or (if it wasn't great), just snuggle up and say "I love being with you."

– **Brave the bottom.** Straight women tend to avoid anal sex. Contrary to popular opinion, not all gay men do it, but they're certainly more open to giving it a go. I've written extensively about the safe way to have anal intercourse in my other books (try *superhotsex*) but here's a reminder of the basics for any anal play: always wash toys before and (obviously) afterward. Use condoms on toys you plan on sharing or using both vaginally and anally. It'll feel more comfortable and be less messy if that high-fiber breakfast has done the trick and if you've had a nice hot shower, swishing lots of soap around your bottom.

Having an orgasm first helps relax the area and using lube is an essential not a pleasure extra. Anal creams that desensitize the anus are not your friend, neither are "poppers" or cocaine. Especially for first-timers. They all do a fantastic job of numbing the area but that's the problem. Pain is nature's warning. Yes, I know that's something your mother would say but there is a right and wrong way to enjoy anal play and pain will tell you which path you're on. If you're not that keen but don't hate it, turn it into a special "treat" for him if he is. (Tight and taboo is an erotic twosome!)

What's hot
Not getting squeamish about sperm. Do gay guys care if it ends up all over them or the newly washed sheets?

What's not
Touching too lightly. It's nice, in a dreamy, tickly way, but men's skin is thicker and tougher. If you're *too* gentle, he won't even feel it.

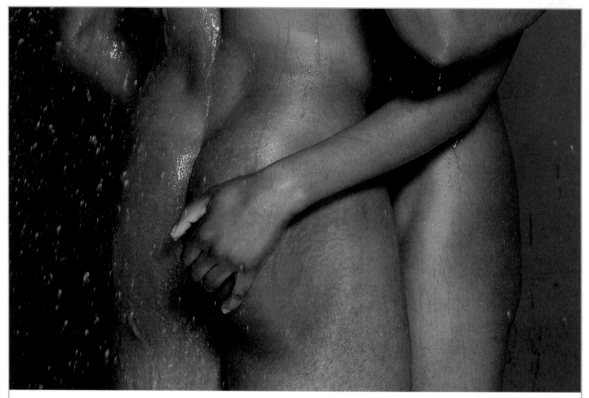

Gay men use lube

Do you want to improve your sex life dramatically—and instantly? Then try using lube. Girls tend to drag it out only for intercourse, gay boys use it for hand-jobs, anal play, during long sessions, with sex toys—for everything!

It even makes safe sex safer: add a drop of lube inside a condom and it's less likely to tear. If you're being ultra-safe and using a dental dam during oral sex, put a tiny amount on your clitoris under the dam and it'll feel so much better.

The trick with lube is getting the amount right. Use too much and you will reduce all friction. So add a little to start with and then top it up rather than overdo it. Which lube is best for what?

Saliva—yours or theirs

This is natural and good for everything. Add some saliva to reactivate lube you added earlier and give it another lease of life.

Household lubes

Hand cream, Vaseline, massage oil, olive oil, and butter work well in movies but not in real life. Some damage condoms, others upset the pH balance of vaginal secretions and cause infections. They can be messy and smelly and a bitch to get out in the wash.

Water-based lubes

These feel and look natural and are great all-rounders. They're safe to use with condoms and toys and come in flavored varieties, so you're not gagging if you end up giving oral after applying one. They're non-irritating and don't stain your sheets or furniture.

Silicone lube

Although it's the most expensive type of lube, it lasts much longer, which means it's the *only* choice for anal sex. Silicone makes it really slippery and it works in water. Be a bit careful though—the clean-up is difficult because it tends to leave a film. Silicone lube sounds like a match made in heaven for silicone sex toys but instead it just damages them so stick to water-based varieties.

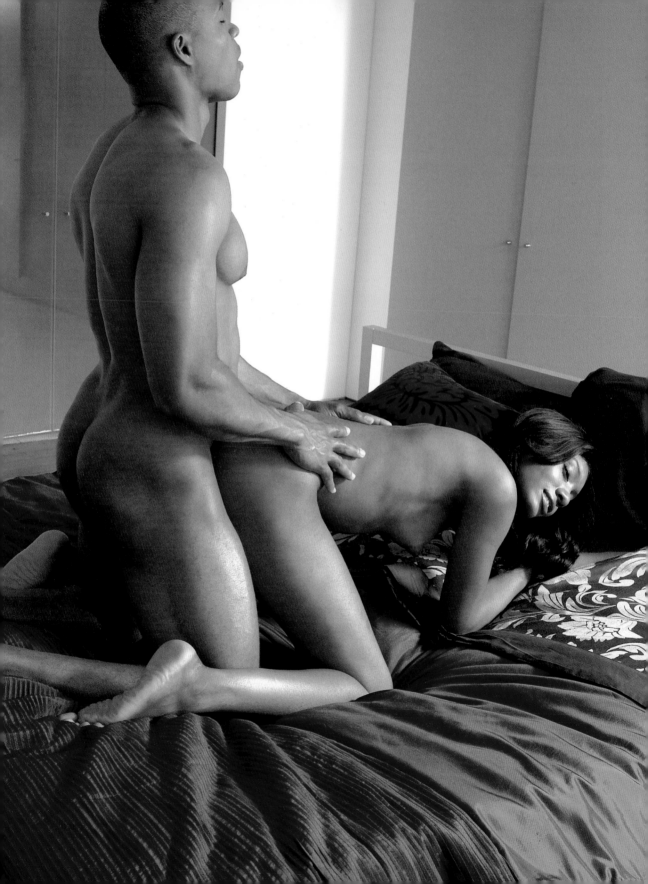

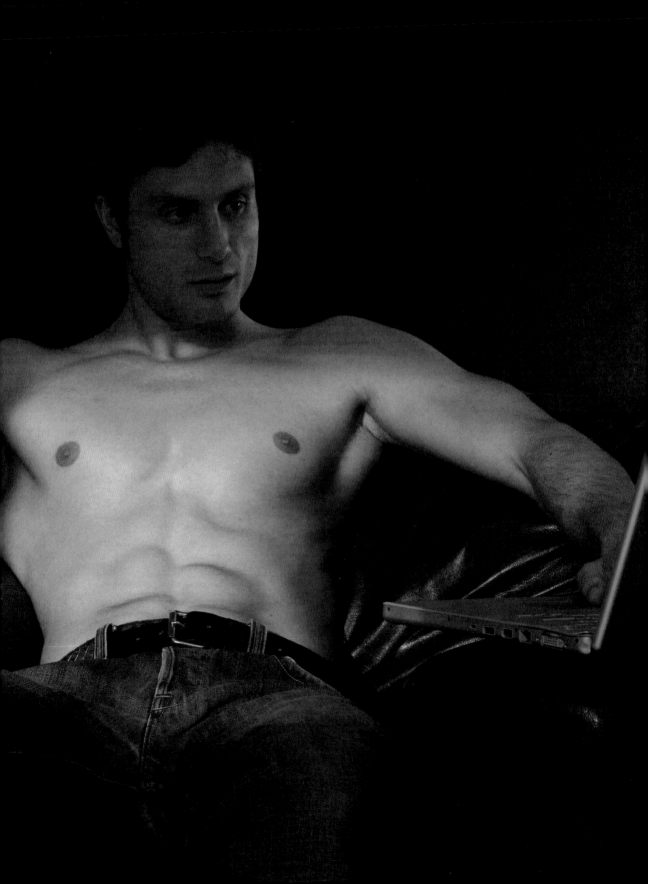

Net Sex: Evil or Erotic?

You'll be an avid fan (usually male) or deeply suspicious (probably female). The truth is, there's good and bad on the net. Here's help on where to point that mouse (among other things) …

The internet has made graphic porn easily available and, like most men, net sex is probably something you do when she's out with the girls. You may decide it's actually preferable to real sex. After all, the girl on screen not only has perkier breasts and a flatter stomach, she'll do just about anything how and when you want it. No wining, dining, talking, compromising, cajoling, or emotional effort required. Just instant, intense visual stimulation, which, when coupled with a practiced DIY hand-job, is a lazy passport to pleasure. Is it any wonder you might be choosing net sex over the real thing?

Research shows the area of the brain that controls emotions and motivation is more activated in men than women when watching erotic images. Given this inborn predilection to porn, should we not just let nature and technology form a natural marriage? Yes—and no. Assuming you use it in moderation, and are an intelligent and emotionally mature man, porn is relatively harmless. It's beneficial in lots of cases. What's not so great, is that internet porn is now how most teenage boys learn about sex. Which has absolutely disastrous consequences.

Think about the lessons to be learned from porn: sex happens with little effort on his part, other than to pull out a ginormous penis. All women moan loudly. Women orgasm effortlessly from just about anything, including often (*owwww*) rough handling of her clitoris or genitals. Women also climax simply by sucking his penis—that's how turned on we are by it. Men get a rock-hard, six-hour erection, whenever they want. He's born knowing what to do. Women like every single thing he does. No one needs to guide anyone or tell them what they need or want. The only talk in bed is dirty talk. STIs don't exist because condoms never make an appearance.

Along with a skewed sense of sexual reality comes an increased risk of sexual addiction. It's on the rise with younger and younger people affected. Experts blame internet porn. Brain research shows behaviors like porn addiction can be just as chemically addictive as drugs and alcohol. Abnormally excessive time and/or money spent surfing porn sites is just as life-debilitating. So that's the really bad news. The good news is that passing up real-life sex for net sex is solvable. And if she checks out "Why Porn Works" (see pages 154–161), she'll find loads of good reasons why you should be exploring internet porn together, rather than chucking your laptop out of the nearest window.

In one US survey, 97 percent of men had accessed internet porn and 2 percent said they'd rather not answer the question. So that's 99 percent then.

1

Net sex is ready when he is—it isn't affected by periods, fat days, moods or arguments. It's predictable—women aren't.

2

It's instant—all he has to do is turn on the computer to turn himself on. No foreplay required.

3

It's lazy sex—most men have a few favorite sites and a particular type of porn they know will push all the right buttons. Zero effort required.

4

It's quick—men are easily aroused by porn because they're visual. He can have a quick solo sex session in the time it takes you to make a cup of coffee.

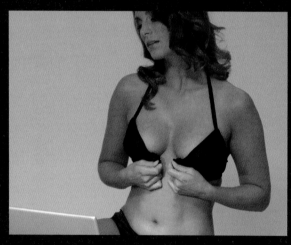

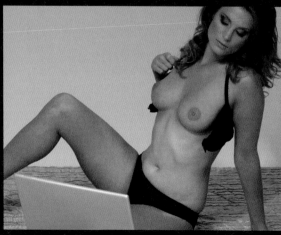

DIY porn

If you can't beat him, join him. Here's how to get involved and enjoy some porn together.

Chatrooms

Why settle for what other, less sexy mortals, have come up with? Customize your porn by visiting a chatroom: there's one for every possible taste. Make up a name and be whoever you want: male, female, bi, gay, straight, old, young, a fantasy profile. Just be aware others are doing the same thing and "hotforitbabe69", who's got you more worked up than you have been in years, could be Bob the plumber, having a laugh. Go on solo or with your partner, seducing each other shamelessly while others watch on in astonishment and envy.

Webcams

Sick of him ogling girls far less sexy than you? There are loads of sites where you can make your own live porn. Be very careful—I'm suggesting more a sneak preview than an I-can-see-what-you-had-for-breakfast type of porn. The idea is you join the site, set up the webcam, send a sexy text message to your partner to link them to the site, and then give them the shock of their life! You don't have to do much other than sit on the bed, look sexy (pretend you're not aware the camera is on), then maybe say, "I'm feeling horny," and take your top off. The thrill is simply seeing you in such a "naughty" environment. You could probably sit there knitting if you wanted to! Later, when you're together, you can watch other couples perform. I wouldn't suggest doing it yourselves unless you honestly don't mind others finding out you'd done it (it's more popular than you think and while your friends/boss/may be just as embarrassed as you to admit seeing you on it, they'll still *know*). You also have to be incredibly sexually secure, with egos as big as your breasts and his penis. People can comment as they're watching you and I know many couples whose sexual confidence has been destroyed by damning net chat.

Cameras

Either take naughty shots of yourself to leave in hiding places for your partner or take provocative pics of each other. Use the self-timer for shots together. Be kind. If the shot looks unflattering through the lens, it's going to look ghastly to your partner. If you or they are self-conscious about a body part, cover it artfully. Take turns and don't get too posed: a little movement looks arty and candid shots usually look better. Lighting is everything—so is using a few standard tricks to make yourselves look good. He needs to stand up straight, flex (everything) and hold his tummy in; she needs to stick out her breasts and bottom, wear heels, and/or point her toes.

Videocams

Think "sex tape" and Paris Hilton probably springs to mind. Now, if she couldn't stop a private tape going public with all those millions, what hope would you have? The risk of letting yourself be filmed having sex is the tape falling into the wrong hands or getting on the internet. The problem is lots of guys—hopefully not the sort sharing your bed—voluntarily go public with the tape because they think it makes them look good. It turns them on letting others see what a "stud" they are or letting them see you in action. It's a common male fantasy to imagine other men making love to their partner. Showing a tape indulges the fantasy without the jealousy part—or the risk his mates will outperform him. Plus he gets that warm, fuzzy feeling that he must be pretty hot, if all his friends want to shag you as well. (Warms the cockles of your heart doesn't it?) If you do want to give it a whirl, insist on exclusive ownership and keep it in a safe place. Or make a tape, watch it, then wipe if off. Or don't even put a tape in the camera. What delivers the kick can be the planning and acting out, rather than watching the end result.

When do I need to worry?

Worried what he's doing while you're curled up in bed reading this book?

– If you've noticed the odd, standard porn site when you (accidentally, of course) click on the history button, don't give it another thought.

– If you do stumble on something he's left behind which isn't garden-variety porn (girl on girl, group sex), it could be a cause for concern. It goes without saying that sex involving children or violence not only warrants a confrontation but a possible call to the police.

– If he's focusing on one particular area—even something relatively innocent like women with enormous breasts—he may end up developing a fetish, where he's unable to become aroused or orgasm without that particular stimulant.

– Other reasons for concern: sex has decreased or stopped but you know he's still having net sex. It's time for a chat ... turn to page 122, for your personal action plan.

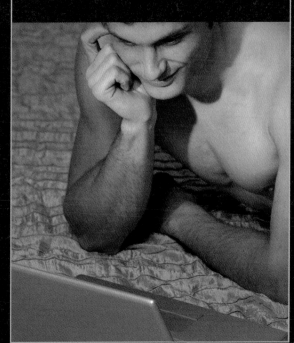

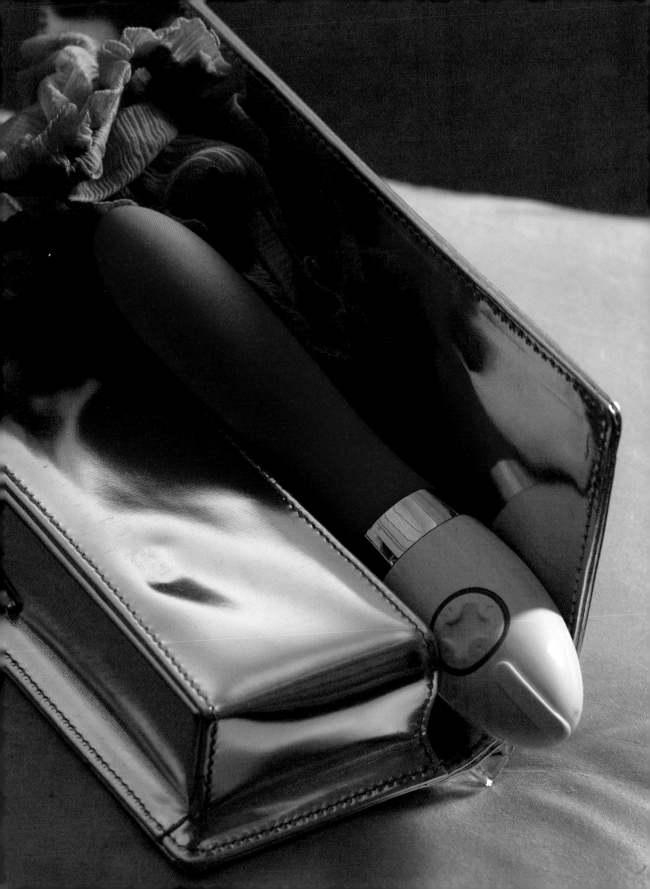

Sex Toys That Work

They're either the best money you ever spent or tossed in the trash after five frustrating minutes. Help on how to choose between a cone, contour, or classic—and whether a butterfly, rabbit, or duck will work for you!

A world without vibrators would be a very, very sad place. So sad, in fact, I think if I stood at the gates of heaven, peered in, and didn't see any, I'd be hot-footing it downstairs. (Especially since downstairs also has lots of forked, lashing tongues!) I suspect I'm not alone. The female fascination with all things that vibrate starts early—as the creators of the now infamous Harry Potter toy broom can testify. An electronic version of the broom, the Nimbus 2000, was invented for children to "ride" around on, presumably pretending they were Harry, off on an exciting adventure. Since it vibrated and was stuck between the legs, young girls had many exciting adventures indeed! (So did Mommy, judging by the glowing reviews.) Sadly, the Nimbus is no longer available. I can't think why ... but I guess those soaring sales tell their own story.

More than one in five adults globally, according to the most recent Durex sex survey, have used a vibrator. Millions are sold each year in most Western countries and the choice is both vast and mind-boggling. Today's vibrators don't just vibrate, they rotate, penetrate, swirl, lick, and seek out parts our parents didn't know existed. They come disguised as bedside lamps, flashlights, lipsticks, cell phones, iPods, and rubber duckies. There are toys for our mouths, bottoms, breasts, nipples, penises, perineums, vaginas, clitorises, and urethras. There are vibrators so small you can lose them in your handbag and so big they look like a rolling pin.

Whenever I take out my old faithful—a rather large "back massager"—from its hiding place, I think of my brother. Not in *that* way, but because he saw it once and when I explained what it was he looked at me with eyes so wide with horror I knew he was thinking "My sister's going to end up in the *Guinness Book of Records* for something I won't want to know about." "Jesus Christ, you could dig up a road with that!" he said. He relaxed a little when I patiently explained it was for external use, but I still see him eyeing me suspiciously now and then.

Apart from possibly my traumatized brother, sex toys are no longer perceived as the pathetic plaything of the "nymphomaniac" (read "a woman who wants sex more than he does"), desperately dateless, or "perverted," They're now so mainstream, any female who doesn't own some type of vibrator is thought of as, well, slightly odd. Sex therapists regularly prescribe vibrators to patients as they remain the easiest, most effective way to bring women to orgasm. Why? The clitoris loves

They're so mainstream, any female who doesn't own some type of vibrator is thought of as slightly odd.

Today's vibrators don't just vibrate, they rotate, penetrate, swirl, lick, and seek out parts our parents didn't know existed.

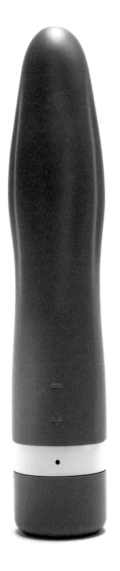

consistent, intense stimulation and *nothing* provides that more efficiently than a vibrator. Hands and tongues don't even get a look in (and penises don't even get a mention). For most women, *nothing*—not even damn good oral sex—can bring us to orgasm quicker than a vibrator. And since the path to orgasm for women is sometimes so bloody long we feel like donning pilgrim sandals and a robe for the journey, anything that speeds up the process isn't appreciated, it's *worshiped*.

Vibrators that work

If you've never had an orgasm, your best possible chance is with a vibrator. If you've never had an orgasm with your partner, the best possible way is to introduce your vibrator into bed with the two of you. If you've never had an orgasm during penetration, it's a vibrator that will get you there. "But, it's my secret!" I can hear you shriek, "I don't think he'd handle it!" I'm with the world famous sexologist Betty Dodson who said if a man can't handle seeing you use a vibrator, keep the vibrator and ditch the man. (For tips on how to broach the topic, see page 118).

As for the suggestion that having orgasms using a vibrator is somehow "cheating," hello! So is wearing mascara! Why do we put our perishables in a fridge rather than stick them in the coolest part of the kitchen, hoping for the best? Because the fridge is about twenty billion trillion times more effective. It's called progress. Yes, you should mix up your orgasm techniques by using your fingers and his tongue but let's not be silly.

Here, I've picked the sex toys that really will improve your sex life—and ignored those that are terrific for about five minutes, then end up chucked in the back of a drawer.

Electric massagers
They never, ever run out of power, they're a one-time investment (I've had mine for 15 years), the vibration is steady, consistent, and teeth-chatteringly strong—hell, you can even pretend it really is for your shoulders! The only negative is that some people freak out because you plug them into the wall. I don't get it. We hold steaming hot hair straighteners with bare hands and apply them perilously close to our scalp and ears and it never occurs to us to worry about being electrocuted. Electric vibrators were invented before irons and vacuum

cleaners! (Good to see someone had their priorities right!) I think they've possibly ironed out any problems by now, don't you? Unless you plug it in while in the tub, you will not electrocute yourself. The Hitachi Magic Wand is the most popular vibrator in the world. If women were mysteriously dying in their bedrooms, legs askew, their vibrator lying beside them, I think we'd have heard about it by now. For fabulous external genital stimulation or if you secretly feel a bit smutty using sex toys, this reassuringly medical-looking number can't be beaten.

Bullet vibes

They look like large tampons, are often made of metal, and sit snugly between the vaginal lips providing strong clitoral stimulation. They're also perfect for caressing nipples, around the rim of your bottom—anywhere you fancy a bit of a buzz. Add perfect portability, sleek, and sexy designs—it's no wonder they're a bestseller.

Classic or "torpedo"-shaped vibes:

These are the cheap, nasty, plastic things you used to find rolling around in your Mom's beside table—slim, cylindrical with a rounded top—but now they look and perform way better. They're cheap, the shape gives a strong vibration and, best of all, they're couple friendly. They're small (but look enough like a penis for him to convince himself this is her idea of the "perfect" penis size) and fairly non-intrusive to hold between you and on her clitoris during sex, but big enough to hit the target.

Best of the rest ...

– **Contour vibes** fit in the palm of your hand and are curved to cover more of the labial area. They're gentle, discreet in shape, and suit a sensitive clitoris.

– **The rabbit** is still one of the most popular vibes, even if most women just use the clitoral attachment. It's a shame when the shaft works so hard, whirling in dizzy circles, to provide maximum vaginal enjoyment, while the rabbit "ears" vibrate madly to tickle your clitoris.

– **Finger vibes** are a great option for a solo "quickie" orgasm whenever and wherever you feel like it, plus they're non-intrusive and non-threatening for him.

– **Butterfly vibrators with harnesses** are ingenious. A small vibrator nestles inside a jelly butterfly-shaped sleeve. Position this on top of your clitoris then use the straps, which go around both legs, to hold it in place. The butterfly wings flutter over your clitoris. It's hands-free so can be left in place during intercourse.

– **U-shaped rocking vibrators** are for girlies who like penetration, G-spot stimulation, and clitoral stimulation simultaneously. You insert the curved end and aim toward your G-spot; the other ridged end sits close to your clitoris, allowing the little bullet vibe on the end to do its stuff. Rock it back and forth using your palm.

– **G-spot vibes and dildos** are longer than normal and have a curve to get them in just the right spot. You need quite firm pressure to stimulate the area, so some come with a bulbous end or ridge.

– **The Cone**—you sit or squat over it and enjoy vibration over multiple parts. *Brilliant* results, just don't try to walk after. The squatting is inspired but not very comfy.

What we used to use

Oversized "realistic" vibrators (I use the term "realistic" loosely since the originals were made of ghastly, hard, beige plastic with painted on purple veins) that were about 10 in (25 cm) long. Made by men and, I suspect, used only by (gay) men. They're still around but greatly improved, if you fancy one. Why you would beats the hell out of me. Most still look like something Lorena Bobbitt left behind.

Our new favorites

Bullet-shaped vibrators, butterflies, rabbits, the Cone—lots designed by women for clitoral stimulation.

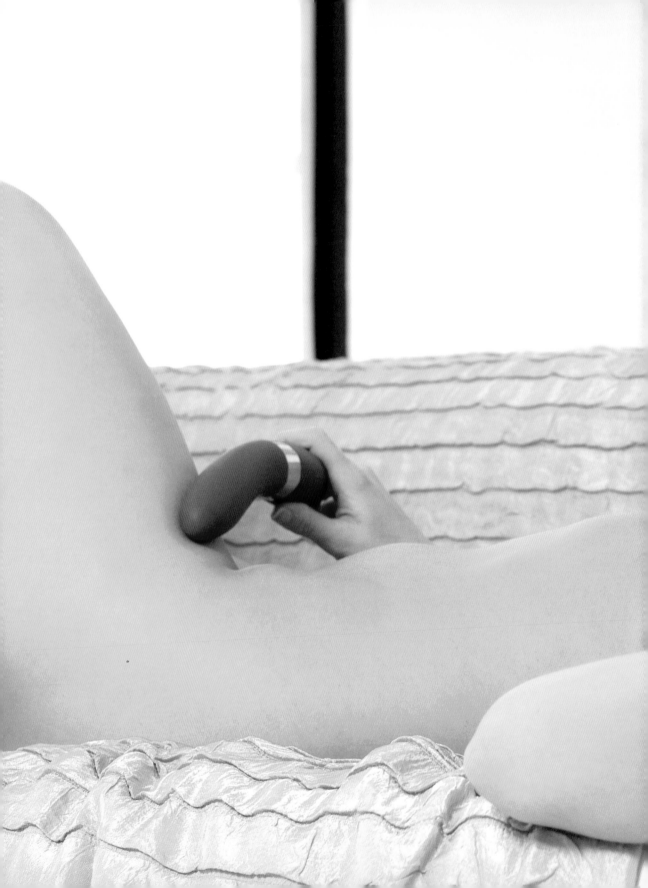

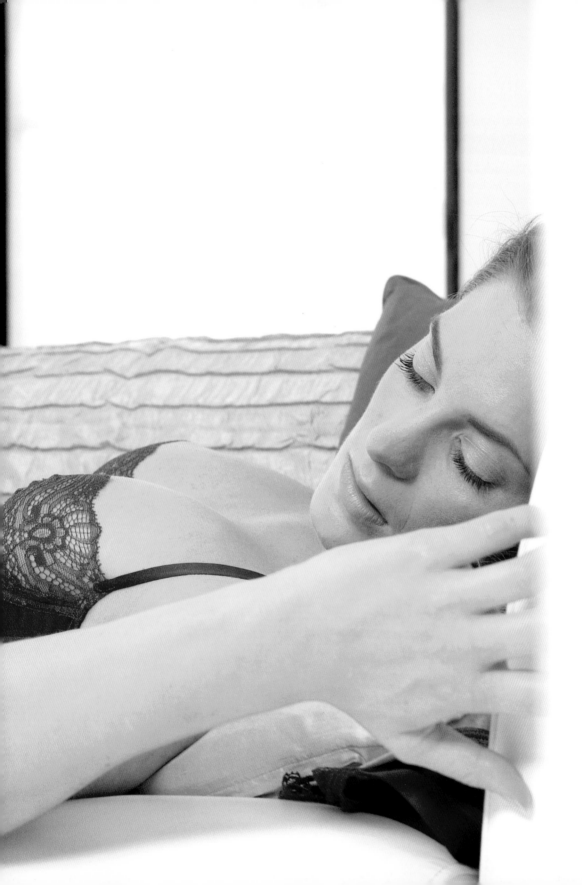

How to buy a vibrator

What do you want to use it for?
The shape depends on whether you want penetration or just clitoral stimulation. (Hopefully, I don't need to point out that the ones that look like penises are supposed to go inside.) If you want both simultaneously, try a rabbit or a U-shaped rocking vibrator (see page 139). You may need more than one vibe. If you want it for anal and vaginal penetration, you'll probably need different sizes.

When are you going to use it?
And don't say, "When I feel like having an orgasm." I mean do you want to travel with it (you'd be amazed how much room a rabbit takes and how a cute little bullet slides into your handbag)? Who's going to be within earshot? Does it need to be super-quiet so roommates can't hear it? Do you have kids and need it "disguised"? I'm not a huge fan of "novelty" vibrators designed to look like lipstick but a "back massager" is a good option. Be wary of the top-end designer vibes that are designed to look like pebbles, for example. They look beautiful and some are OK but others have such weak vibration you'd have more orgasms from getting a real pebble out of the garden and rubbing it to and fro.

How strong is it?
Opt for one that's stronger than you need and keep it on low setting. You can calm it down by putting a T-shirt between you and it or hold your hand over to absorb excessive vibration. Here's why: a few drinks doesn't just make your brain pleasantly numb, it does the same to other parts. Nothing more frustrating than tottering home from a great girls' night out to find you can't even feel your vibrator, let alone orgasm from it. That top speed will then come in mighty handy.

How much should you spend?
You can be lucky and pick up a cheap classic vibe for a couple of bucks and have happy endings till you're 80. Some fall apart after two uses. If you use a reputable site, they will refund your cash if you aren't happy. (You can try any of my range at www.traceycox.com and return them if you don't like them, for instance.) Otherwise, I'd stick to one of the top four faves—bullet, classic, massager, or rabbit – and buy the best you can afford. Apart from batteries, it's a one-off cost and what price can you put on a lifetime of effortless orgasms?

Bottom toys that won't make you run away

Even those who enjoy a finger up their bottom, often baulk at the thought of an anal sex toy. But there's nothing less threatening—and cuter—than the unisex butt plug. Why would you want one?

- Well, instead of inserting that finger and losing the use of a whole hand that could be doing other stuff, the butt plug goes in and stays in. So you've got hands and fingers to put in other pies.

- Some plugs vibrate to tease the anus's ultra-sensitive nerve endings, others sit there quietly but no less effectively by using pure pressure.

- Butt plugs and anal dildos have flared ends or a base. You don't have to be a doctor in a hospital emergency ward to figure out why.

- Don't forget it's essential that you use lube with anal toys because the rectum isn't self-lubricating. And try to use the high-quality, long-lasting stuff, please.

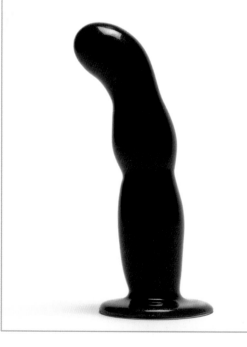

Where to buy them?

Going to a sex shop is a giggle but for the best selection, price, and privacy, go online. If you can't wait, pop to a department store, stand beside the nice lady deciding which toaster to buy and innocently pick up a gloriously powerful "back massager."

Dildos that do the job

The main difference between a phallic-shaped vibrator and a dildo is dildos usually don't vibrate. (If they do, they really belong in the vibrator category.) Dildos are designed for vaginal and anal penetration (see left).

Some women buy them and insert them while using a vibrator on their clitoris but very few use one solo. They're nearly always used in conjunction with a tongue, fingers, or a penis (if it's inserted anally). There's lots of dildo girl-on-girl action in porn but all the gay girls I know say they're no different than straight women—some love being penetrated, others aren't that into it. The big plus about dildos is that you can create your perfect penis because they're sold by width and length. Difficult to find the perfect penis attached to the perfect man in the real world but not in Dildo Land. They're also what you'd buy if your boyfriend wants to be penetrated, in which case buy a model with a harness so you can strap it on.

DIY dildos are everywhere. In your bathroom (the end of a hairbrush), in the fridge (zucchinis, cucumbers, carrots), and the fruit bowl (remove the scratchy bit from the banana end and make sure it's underripe). Peel veggies to the perfect size, and wash them or pop on a condom to protect yourself from pesticides if you don't buy organic.

Dildos can also be put in mouths but usually aren't for obvious reasons. First up, the dildo is unlikely to orgasm. Secondly, they taste bloody awful.

Keep it clean

Follow these guidelines to stay safe:

— Always store sex toys separately from each other because some deteriorate if in direct contact. Buy some cheap cloth shoe bags to put them in, rather than plastic.

— Check the packaging for special instructions before throwing it out. If you don't have the instructions, go online to check them.

— Pop a condom on a sex toy for no-fuss clean-up if you're sharing toys or intend using a toy both anally and vaginally.

— Baby wipes are brilliant to quickly wipe toys off straight after use (and for cleaning up after sex in general).

— Soft, porous toys made of cyberskin, jelly, or rubber can usually be scrubbed or washed with soap and water. Use a "soap-free" or non-alkaline wash if you're prone to thrush. Always rinse and dry them thoroughly.

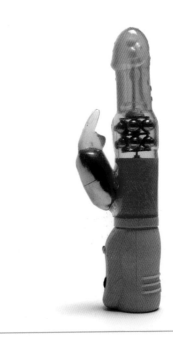

If you want the prettiest one, go for glass. Some of the colored ones are so gorgeous, you'll want it on your coffee table. As a decoration as well, I mean.

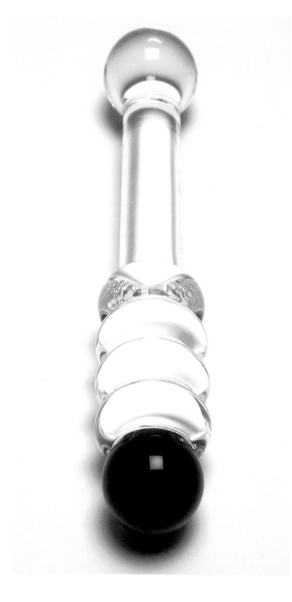

How to buy a dildo

How big do I want it?
They're measured by diameter (across) and length. The most popular lengths are 6 in (15 cm) for standard vaginal penetration; or 8 in (20 cm)—try this size if you're aiming for your front vaginal wall and/or G-spot.

How do I want it to feel inside?
Porous dildos are made of softer materials like latex rubber. They feel nicer but you need to be super-scrupulous about cleaning them. Non-porous dildos (glass, hard plastic, silicone) don't feel "natural" because they're hard—but the upside is they're smooth, so there are less places for nasty bacteria to gather. You'll also get the strong pressure needed for G-spot and anal orgasms from acrylic and plastic dildos.

If you want the prettiest one, go for glass. Some of the colored ones are so gorgeous, you'll want it on your coffee table. As a decoration as well, I mean. Glass lasts a lifetime (so long as you don't drop it), it's easy to keep clean (pop it in the dishwasher), and there's no such thing as a glass allergy. Jelly dildos are fun and cheap but don't expect them to be around longer than your current real-life toy boy. Cyberskin dildos feel *uncannily* real but, again, be prepared to do the washing-up afterward.

How am I going to use it?
– **Some dildos have suction caps** that secure them to a surface so you can squat over them.

– **You can also get double-ended dildos**, if you like feeling "full" in your anus and vagina during solo sex or want to use it with a partner. Each end for each girl's vagina if you're lesbian, one end in her vagina, the other in his anus if you're straight, and one end in each guy's anus if you're gay. (Confused?)

– **Dildos can also be put in mouths** but usually aren't for obvious reasons. First up, the dildo is unlikely to orgasm. Secondly, they taste bloody awful. Flavored condoms are OK but I don't know anyone who'd put one in their mouth just for the hell of it.

– **Strap-on dildos** are worth investing in if you like using a dildo. Why? They free up your hands so you can use them to simultaneously stimulate other areas.

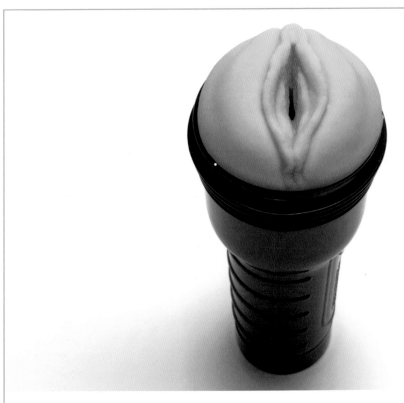

Boys' toys

Nearly all the sex toys for her—vibrators, anal toys, etc—can conceivably be used on him as well (his testicles, perineum, anus). But then there are those designed *just* for men.

The Fleshlight

This is a shining example of a boys' toy. Shaped like a flashlight (hence the fleshlight pun), it's a masturbation sleeve that uses creepily realistic cyberskin to create a fake mouth, vagina, or anus. He puts his penis where the light doesn't shine, entering a 10in- (25cm-) deep sleeve (yes, it was invented by a man—an ex LA cop who based the design on the US cop's standard flashlight!).

The inside is completely customized. It can be smooth or ridgy and however tight he wants it. He thrusts in and out the sleeve and before he can exclaim "How easy is this!", it's not only provided a rather satisfying orgasm, it does the cleaning-up afterward (semen neatly collects in the end). The Fleshlight is conveniently both washable and reusable. With Fleshlights and rabbits (see page 139) around, it's hard to believe we're still even bothering with this whole relationship thing!

Prostate massagers

These look like something you'd pick up off the surface of the moon—they are odd, alien-shaped objects that he inserts up his rectum to stimulate the many nerve endings inside the anus. Some prostate massagers vibrate, some don't.

Sex dolls

You can buy anything from a clone of your favorite porn star to, well, a girl with big breasts, long legs, and long hair. (Spot the difference.) The plastic dolls you see blokes carrying around on stag nights cost about ten quid. Fork out around $400 and you can buy creepily realistic models, made from surgical latex, that have a mouth begging to eat you and a bottom and vagina that vibrate. (For God's sake, guys, don't even think about it. How on earth is a real-life girl ever going to compete after that?)

Bite Eat Nibble
Scratch Suck
Lick Taste Grab
Grind Thrust
Deep Hard
Swallow Ravish
Shag Screw
Tight Erect Stiff
Come Orgasm
Tease Touch
Fondle Push Pull
Slap Pinch Juicy
Hot Soft Throb
Horny Wet
Hungry Open
Need Want Big

The Other Oral Sex

How do I tell my lover what I'd like without offending them? I want to talk dirty but what the hell do I say? They're two of the questions I'm asked the most often—and, guess what? The answers, and everything you always wanted to know about sex talk, are right here.

When you're shagging yourselves silly in the early days of your relationship, talking about sex is easy. In fact, most of us don't shut up about it. We're all smug and self-congratulatory about how naughty we are, how hot the other person is, how our friends are jealous that we can't keep our hands off each other, blah, blah, blah. It's only when things go wrong that we clam up. Not so much fun talking about sex when you're not up for it, not having it, or don't enjoy doing it.

But here's the deal: if you can't talk about sex with your partner, you aren't going to be having it long-term. Kid yourself all you want that the odd grunt, groan, or moan is all you need to communicate lust. That the six-year sex rut you're in will just fix itself with time. That your husband's wandering eye has nothing to do with the fact that you haven't slept with him for a year. That your wife's yoga lesson really does go on till 10pm. That if you concentrate hard enough, he'll finally figure out where your clitoris is. Dream on. Talking about sex doesn't just fix these problems, it reassures us, deepens trust, and makes us feel "normal." It creates desire, titillates, and—

most importantly of all—stops us sliding into the perilously tedious, God-do-we-really-have-to sexual doldrums.

With so many advantages to talking about sex, why don't we do it? Because if you choose the *wrong* words, the opposite can happen. You can just as easily upset, deflate, and devastate your partner, destroying what little sex life you had left. No wonder we're all so nervous about opening up to each other. Now I've really got your attention, let's look at how you and your partner can open the channels of communication—and inject some seriously spicy sex into your life.

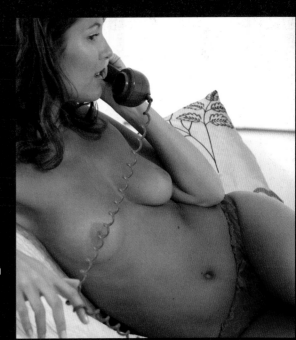

Start talking

Yes, you really must have a "We're going to talk about sex" conversation. Start by shaking on it to make it an official deal. Set ground rules: agree not to judge each other. Agree not to get all huffy and sulky if one of you confesses the other's signature swirly tongue "it worked on a supermodel" technique actually doesn't do it for you. Set yourselves up for open, honest communication. This means compliments but also (constructive) criticism.

Firstly, have a chat

– **Know what you want.** This sounds basic but lots of people don't know. Be specific. You want more sex? How much more? What type—intercourse, oral, hand-jobs? When do you want it? Where? For how long *exactly*? Which part do you want to last the longest? Do you want more orgasms or sex more often or for it to last longer? Really think things through before you talk.

– **Be selective.** Decide how much of your past you want to share. Some people are curious and amused hearing about the lesbian experiments you had when you were in college, and how your last ex made weird grunting noises when he came. Others don't want to know any details about any past lovers because all it does is set up a full-color videotape that whirls around and around in their head—and not in a good way.

– **Agree you can stop new things *at any time*.** One of my friends was told "Stop, this isn't working for me" two seconds after he'd penetrated. Two minutes later the girl had her clothes on and was out the door. He was left sitting on the bed in shock. Now *that* took guts. While this is an extreme example and I don't suggest for a second you do the same (I've been consoling the guy ever since), it's pointless pretending you're enjoying something if you're not. It takes courage to say, "This isn't actually doing it for me" 15 minutes into an elaborate roleplay, but even if that Princess Leia outfit will hang, forlorn and unworn, in the wardrobe, you're still wise to speak up. If you know you can say no after you've started, it will encourage you both to try stuff you're pretty convinced *you* won't like, but know puts a glint in your partner's eye. Having said that, if your partner's really getting into it and you're so-so but not hating it, indulge them for a little while longer.

Good things to say and try

– Do you like it when I do it here/ hard/soft/like this/like that?
– I love licking you.
– Which way do you like it best— like this or that?
– Your ass is so divine. Do you want me to spank it?
– Do you want me to put a finger inside you?
– Can I kiss you here?

Never ever say or do

– I hate it when you do that.
– John used to do this with his fingers.
– Shout "And you're bad in bed!" in the middle of an argument.
– Say "Why don't we ever do this or that?" in an accusatory voice.
– Demand rather than ask.

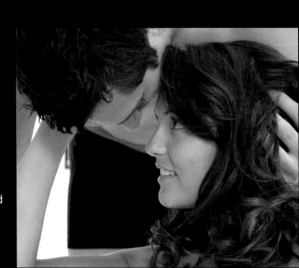

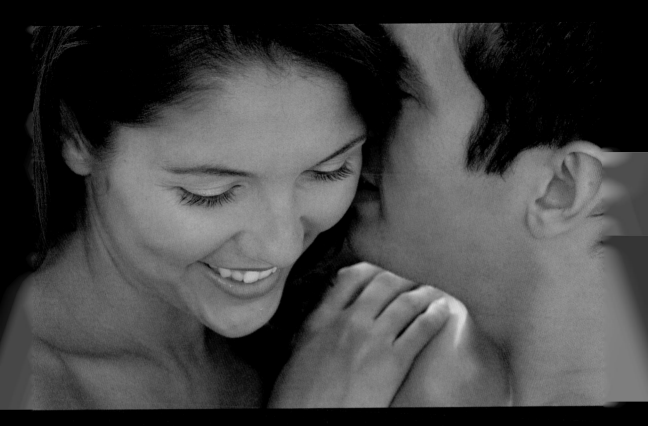

Share any past traumatic sex experiences. I'm not suggesting you launch into a confession about the time you walked in on your sister and a cucumber, but in a long-term relationship it is necessary to share. If some guy forced you to give him oral sex in college, that'll explain why you're not falling to your knees the second he waves his erect penis in the air. People don't mind you saying no if they understand why and it gives them a good idea what's out of bounds. It's not necessary short-term but is for true intimacy.

Now do it

Tell and show each other your hot spots—and discover new ones. Spend one session licking, stroking, biting, caressing (you get the picture) each other *everywhere*. Who'd have thought a tongue swishing between your toes would feel so good? We forget things. I love having my neck bitten but one guy I went out with hated doing it. Thought it was barbaric (which was sort of the point, you can see why that one didn't last!). I'd forgotten how much I loved it until the next lover ventured there. Also remember, hot spots change over time (second by second, if we're talking

Compliment each other. Say how hot they look, how good they are at certain things. Do it often. This is the one time you won't get in trouble for repeating yourself.

Be responsive. If your partner tentatively tries something, respond. We're all a little bit shy, so if you notice she gives your bottom an experimental slap or he holds your hands together above your head, react for God's sake! Either say a very obvious "*Ummmm*" at the time or "Hey, that was hot, what you did" afterward. Nothing worse than working up the courage to try something and then having no idea whatsoever if the person noticed, liked it, or hated it!

Do your research. You've bought this book (thanks, by the way), so *share* what you've learnt with your partner. Try it out. Buy at least one or two good sex books a year to keep up on new techniques and to give you imaginative new things to try. Flip through them and note things you'd like to give a whirl.

Feed desire. Read erotic books, try porn. Talk about it together, read out bits. Show each other sexy stuff

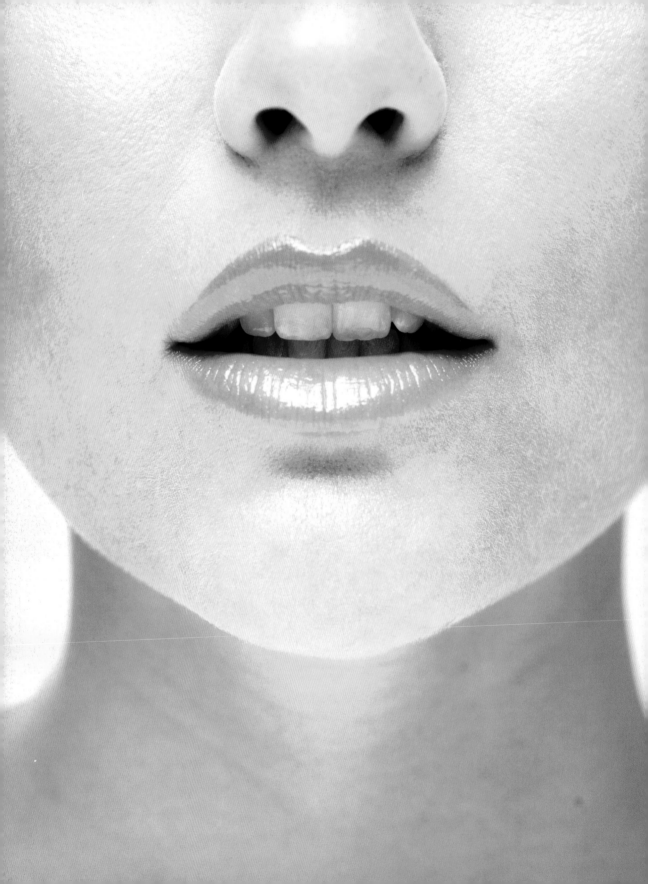

If you don't ask, you don't get …

- **If you want more of the same,** talk to your partner about the great times you've already had in bed. Say exactly what you loved about it ("Wasn't it great to make love outside?"). It builds up a partner's confidence and cements your sexual history. Couples who talk a lot about the good times they've had tend to be happier than those who don't.

- **If you want something done differently,** gently suggest new things, rather than criticize what your partner's already doing. So try saying, "I love it when you give me oral. Can you do it for longer, sometimes I feel rushed," rather than saying, "You never give me oral sex for long enough."

- **If you want to try a new position,** pick up a good positions sex book (my *Kama Sutra* has got enough to keep you both happy for a year!). Each go through it and mark the positions you'd like to try. Then read the written instructions, look at the picture, and put yourselves into position.

- **If you want him to use your vibrator** on you during intercourse, start by suggesting a vibrating penis ring. He wears it over his penis, giving the illusion it's his huge, manly member doing the trick, rather than the craftily placed little vibrator working its magic on your clitoris. (Just make sure he grinds in a circular fashion, maintaining good contact between the vibe and you, or it really will just be down to his penis alone.) Bullet vibrators are great for "lodging" in place between the vaginal lips while he penetrates and butterfly vibes are also easy to ignore.
See Sex Toys That Work, pages 136–145, and Instant Sex Makeovers, page 118, for other tips.

- **If you have a fantasy you want to share** with your partner during sex, consider taping it and turning it on as you start to have sex. Mouths are (and should be) kept busy during a good sex session, making it hard to talk. If you want to use the fantasy as a mood-setter, send it to your partner via email or feed it through, bit by bit, by text. One crucial tip before acting on this one: make it very clear what you want done with the fantasy.

Is it just to turn the two of you on? Do you want to roleplay (see below)? Or actually do it in reality? All are very, very different things.

- **If you want to suggest something a bit "out there",** try renting a movie that showcases what you want to do in an appealing way (*9½ Weeks* for tie-ups and ice-cubes; *The Secretary* for B&D). Watch their reaction while it's on. If they look intrigued, say "That's sexy. I wouldn't mind some of that ... Do you?" Or buy a book or erotic magazine that features it and leave it lying around. Another old favorite—"I had a dream last night we were doing such-and-such ..." and watch to see what their response is.

- **If you want to talk dirty but can't bring yourself to,** make a tape or leave voicemail on their cell phone (never, ever leave it on their answer machine at home—we've all seen the sitcoms), write a sexy email, send a text or instant message, leave a note in their pocket or wallet, hell, write a message on the mirror in the steam from the shower. Or call them at work when you know they can't answer back and tell them exactly what you've got planned for that night. "Just thought you'd like to know I'm masturbating right now because I can't wait to be inside you later," then hang up.

- **If you want to roleplay** but know it's not their "thing," try adding subtle props that trigger the fantasy for you, so your partner doesn't feel like they're in some cheesy B-grade porn movie. He leaves his shirt on and suddenly becomes the hot door-to-door salesman. The gorgeous garter belt and stockings you bought her "just because" nicely indulge the "she's a sex worker, I'm the client" fantasy.

Agree not to get all huffy if one of you confesses the other's signature swirly tongue "it worked on a supermodel" technique actually doesn't do it for you.

Talking dirty

Just like before, set some ground rules to find out what would turn both of you on.

Have the chat

- **What sort of language do you want to use?** Set limits if one of you doesn't like slang or swear words. (Be careful with emotionally charged phrases like "You're a dirty slut." Some women love it because it's so politically incorrect, others find it insulting.)

- **When should you do it?** Just before orgasm or to get you in the mood? What about if she whispered in your ear in public?

- **What sort of themes?** (You're a slut, you're a virgin, you're a goddess). Do you want a beginning, middle, and end to it—more a fantasy than dirty talk?

- **How do you want it?** Do you want it soft and sexy, low and sinister, forceful and disrespectful? Do you want them to say stuff, but for you not to answer?

- **Do you want to pretend you're other people?** Some people love pretending their partner's "sleeping" with someone else, others get jealous, which destroys the mood in two minutes flat, and leads to discussions like "This is about John, isn't it! He's got blonde hair and bulging muscles. You're fantasizing about him!"

Now do it

- **Pitch your voice lower than usual.** If you're shy, whisper in their ear so there's no eye contact or try blindfolding them, or letting them blindfold you.

- **Keep it simple to start.** Describe what he's doing to you. "You've got your hands on my breasts." Add what that makes you feel, "... And it feels wonderful."

- **Describe what you're doing or about to do.** "I'm going to take your penis in my mouth and suck it." Add what that makes you feel—"... And it makes me feel powerful. Like you're in my control."

- **Compliment body parts.** Tell your partner "I love your muscles," or "You've got the best ass I've ever seen." Pause, draw back, and let your eyes totally devour what's in front of you, then look them straight in the eye and say "You're beautiful. I want you so much." Talk about how good you are together—"God, I so love our sex together."

- **Encourage dirty talk.** Ask "Do you like that?", "What does it feel like?", "Do you want more?", "What would you like me to do to you now? I'll do anything ..."

- **Let them know where you're at arousal-wise.** "Ummm, this is starting to feel really nice", or "God, I'm so close to coming."

- **Let her know how much you want to please her,** "I'm going to make you come so hard, you won't know what's happened."

- **Let him know how good he looks**—"I love watching your face when you come." Give a blow-by-blow description—"Your tongue feels amazing. That's just amazing. Keep doing it. Don't stop."

- **Read aloud something sexy** from a book or a magazine while your partner works on you.

- **Pay attention to body language.** Just because your partner isn't saying anything or is coyly refusing to look you in the eye, doesn't mean they're not enjoying it! Is he getting harder? Is she getting wetter? Are they breathing harder? You're doing fine, so keep going.

- **Give cunningly disguised direction.** "Use that gorgeous wet tongue to lick me right there. Really soft. Get it really wet. Swish it around. Just like that."

Some women love to scream obscenities at the top of their voice and don't care if the neighbors change lines at the supermarket checkout.

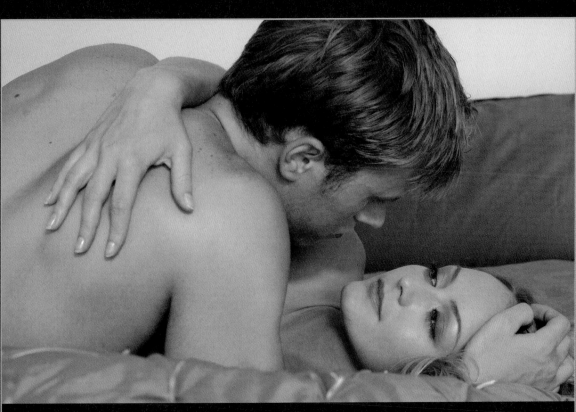

Why talking dirty makes us nervous?

Again, it's so, so easy in the beginning. You'd eyeball them suggestively and ask them to do things Angelina Jolie would have blushed at. (That's back in the Billy Bob days rather than Mother Teresa reinvent.) It's later, when you're mates, that it just starts to feel wrong somehow. Incestuous. You're not alone—it's normal to feel more embarrassed talking dirty as time goes on, rather than the reverse. But, like most things in sex, all you need to fix it is to actually start doing it again—and challenge any negative thoughts.

It's taboo

Parents who taught us sex was "bad," religious beliefs, a past lover who branded you "unladylike" (read slutty)—all make us nervous about speaking up. Beat it. Tell your partner why it's hard for you to talk dirty and that you need to take baby steps. Give yourself permission—parents don't know everything, you can be spiritual and still have great sex, your past lover had serious issues. Try saying naughty things out loud to yourself first. Practice in front of a mirror at first.

You're scared you'll laugh

Yes you will. Talking dirty is funny. That's why you have to do it when you're both turned on because the second you've climaxed, whatever you or your partner just said seems either hilarious or really perverted. So don't freak out when it happens, just keep going.

You don't know what to say

Some women love screaming obscenities at the top of their voice and don't care if the neighbors change lines at the supermarket checkout. Others don't like slang and swear words and that's OK! Whispering "I want you. Now" can be just as erotic (to some men, more so!). So don't try to be something you're not. On the other hand, if your partner shoots through the roof if you use "dirty" words, indulge them. Come up with some compromises: he wants you to use the nasty "C" word, you don't. How about "pussy"? Come on, that's the word you call your cat!

Why Porn Works

Women love it just as much as men do. But how do you suggest watching something saucy, how do you choose from a scary selection of carnal cheese, and what the hell do you do while you're watching it, apart from look highly embarrassed and laugh?

My last boyfriend had never, ever watched porn with a girl so I decided that had to be fixed instantly. "Should I buy some?" he asked, biting his lip and looking a bit nervous. "No, I've got loads!" I boasted. "We'll do it when you come over tonight." Nudge nudge, wink wink. So he arrives at my place, a spring in his step and a glint in his eye and I go to the cupboard to get out my porn stash ... and realize it's all on videotape. Which makes me look about as hip as Pat Boone. Second problem: I don't own a video player. Great.

Frantically searching through my DVDs for something, *anything* (hell, a hot version of *The Sound of Music* would have done at that point), my feverish fingers finally stumbled upon a DVD that might just do the trick. A really old instructional lovemaking DVD. "What's that?" my boyfriend asked suspiciously. "It looks educational." "It's more sexy than educational," I lied, nose growing like Pinocchio while my boyfriend's extendable part seemed to be moving in the opposite direction.

But we put the DVD on and started watching and snogging. Even I had to admit it was a bit lame but when the narrator said, "If a man puts his penis inside the vagina he'll feel intense pleasure," my boyfriend couldn't take it any longer. Right in the middle of giving me (rather good) oral sex, he burst out laughing. "Who is this stuff for? Like, who can't work that one out?' So then we went to Blockbuster but no porn there, then we tried an adult satellite channel but it didn't start till 8pm. In desperation, we got the laptop out and went online but by the time we'd chosen a film, the bloody battery gave out and who designed computer power cords so short you can't plug the thing in and prop it up to watch and have sex at the same time? So we gave up.

Your experience, however, will be fabulous! (First tip—never promise what you can't deliver. The second – always come prepared. If you want to come at all.) Millions and millions of "normal" people rent, buy, download, and watch porn every year. The industry is worth billions. Men watch it, women watch it, couples watch it. It's thought about half the sales and rentals of porn DVDs are to females—though while they tend to use it with their partners, men use theirs to masturbate. Just like anal sex, porn jumped over the "kinky" fence to become mainstream a few years ago.

But one final thing before you press play: remember female porn stars are cast for their vulvas and their breasts. Prepare yourself for pink, symmetrical, hairless, pretty little things with inner lips smaller than the outer lips. Men are hired for their penis size, staying power, and ability to effortlessly get an erection and ejaculate on cue. Both sexes are hired for their ability to have lots of sex with no apparent wear and tear. One female porn star called Houston allegedly had sex with 621 men in under eight hours. Your body and genitals probably don't look or work like theirs. Just thought you might like to know.

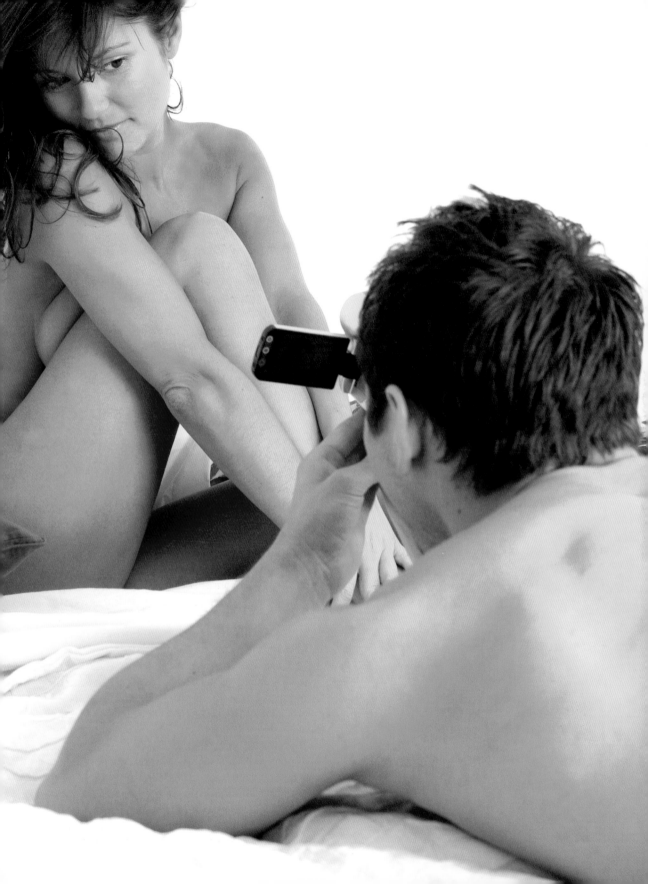

If perfect porn chicky-babes are the *only* girls you watch and fantasize about, it will interfere with real-life sex.

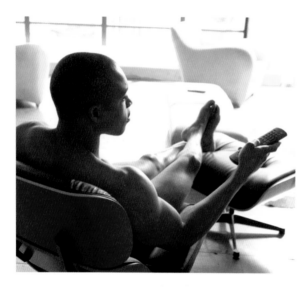

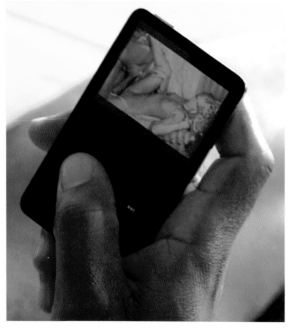

Tuning in together

How to suggest it

If you're used to talking about sex openly, suggesting to your partner you watch a porn flick together isn't a big deal. If you're a little shy, see pages 148–151. Most people are curious, if a tad apprehensive, and the trick to talking them into it is usually just using the right bait. One Dutch study found women responded positively to porn made by women and negatively to male-made porn, without being told which was which. Gosh, wonder why that'll be then? Could it have something to do with the fact that the women in the female-directed porn *didn't* have huge breasts (silicone), long blonde hair (extensions), perfect bodies (surgery, genes), and equally perfect genitals (surgery—lots of porn stars get their labia trimmed and clitoris enlarged so they look pink and lean. Hell, one porn star got cheek implants so she'd look good in blow-job shots!).

I'm not being bitchy here (well …) just pointing out that these girls weren't born looking like this. So it's silly to beat yourself up about not looking like them (if, indeed, you'd want to). If you're eager to give porn a try, but don't want to feel suicidal about your looks, opt for films that advertise "naturals" (no surgery). Or go for amateur" porn, where cellulite and stretch marks abound!

How to choose it

Female porn is less explicit and a really good place to start for *anyone*—male or female. Far less in-your-face. Literally. If your partner says they've tried porn but hated it, it usually means they've watched hard-core porn and didn't like it. Having said that, our taste in porn is as individual as we are. Luckily, there's so much out there, I defy anyone not to find something they like. Where to start? Why not try a mainstream film that has sex in it? *Basic Instinct* for brilliant bondage, *Henry and June* for girl-on-girl, *The Secretary* for spanking and S&M, *Eyes Wide Shut* for voyeurism, *The Piano* for "a bit of rough."

– **Turn up the heat** if that (or you) go down well, by renting more obvious sex films like *Emmanuelle*, *The Story of O*, *Wild Orchid*, and *Lady Chatterley's Lover*. Or turn on the porn channel in a hotel—it's guaranteed to be soft-core. The next step is to go online, Google "free porn" and prepare to be utterly overwhelmed by the astonishing selection of porn available at no cost.

Good reasons to watch porn

– It's fun.

– It gets us off quickly.

– It's great to masturbate to.

– It's something different to do.

– You're voyeurs.

– You're both confident sexually and physically, and your partner makes you feel so attractive you'd never be threatened by what's on screen.

– It's naughty.

– It stops you from feeling left out if he watches it without you.

– It can make it easier to talk about sex.

– It provides a sneak preview of stuff you might like to try.

– Explicit visual stimulation is a key factor for long-term desire.

Good reasons not to watch

– If you've got a bad body image.

– If you have concerns about your genital appearance or size.

– If you're insecure in your relationship.

– If you just don't feel sexy right now.

– If your partner doesn't make you feel attractive.

– If he's a premature ejaculator.

– If he's having erection problems.

– If there's a history of sexual abuse.

You'll find what's on offer for free is usually divided into categories such as girl-on-girl, group sex, and amateur. Find the category you like most. The drawback with free porn is that you only get about three minutes worth. Plenty of time to (ahem) "watch and wank" but not enough to enjoy together. Your choice then is to download a longer version or buy or rent a DVD from one of the many adult sites. For porn with a bit of passion, I'd stick with female directors or independent or amateur films.

– **Some recommendations:** for female directors, some-thing by Anna Span, Tina Tyler, Veronica Hart, or Candida Royalle. There are lots of sites devoted purely to rating porn films. Or read *The Ultimate Guide to Adult Videos* by Violet Blue for a rundown on the best. Ratings wise, Triple XXX is the most explicit, showing penetration, money ("come") shots, and genital close-ups. At the other end are "educational" films.

– **For quirky and sexy,** try *The Nina Hartley Guides*. She's an ex porn star with 650 films under her belt. I met her at a trade exhibition, when she was signing copies of her books. She wasn't hard to find—anyone with a pulse was hanging around, all swoony and kicking the floor like shy schoolboys in the face of such perfection (she's seriously gorgeous!). In her guides, she dispenses sex tips via diagrams and live demonstrations by her "friends." Hilarious but sexy and you can even buy them on Amazon, so there's no embarassing listings on your credit-card statement. (Most adult film suppliers trade under innocuous names for that reason.)

– **Consider getting some gay porn** if you'd prefer to see good-looking men, rather than pretty average guys with enormous penises. The men in gay porn are loads better looking! (Apparently, producers of mainstream porn deliberately choose not-so-great looking men so their main viewer—your average guy—isn't left feeling inadequate. Poor dear.)

Take turns

If you and your partner like different styles of porn, be gracious—no rolling of eyes when it's not your choice. If your partner wants to watch something you're not sure about, watch it solo using fast-forward. You'll know what you're in for and can always close your eyes during the really bad bits!

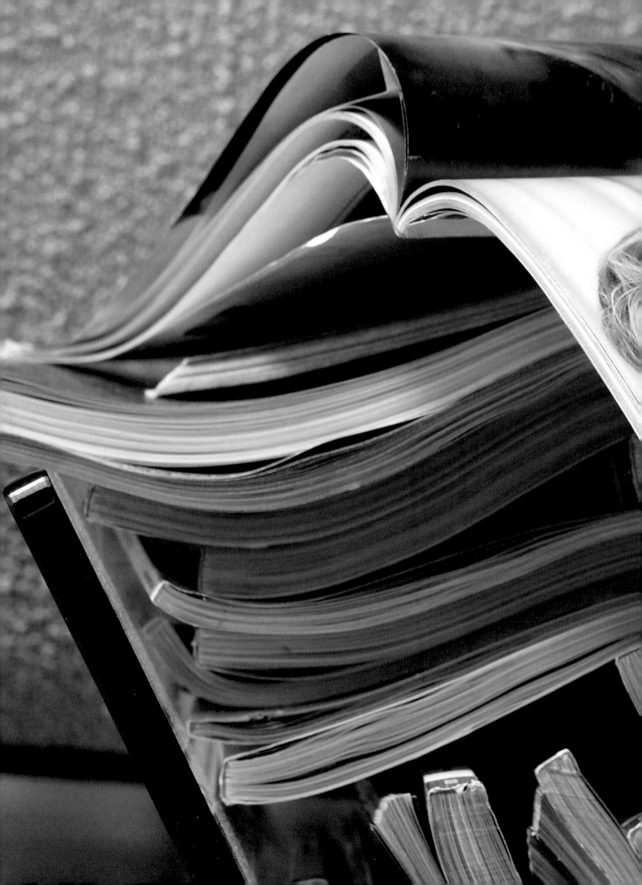

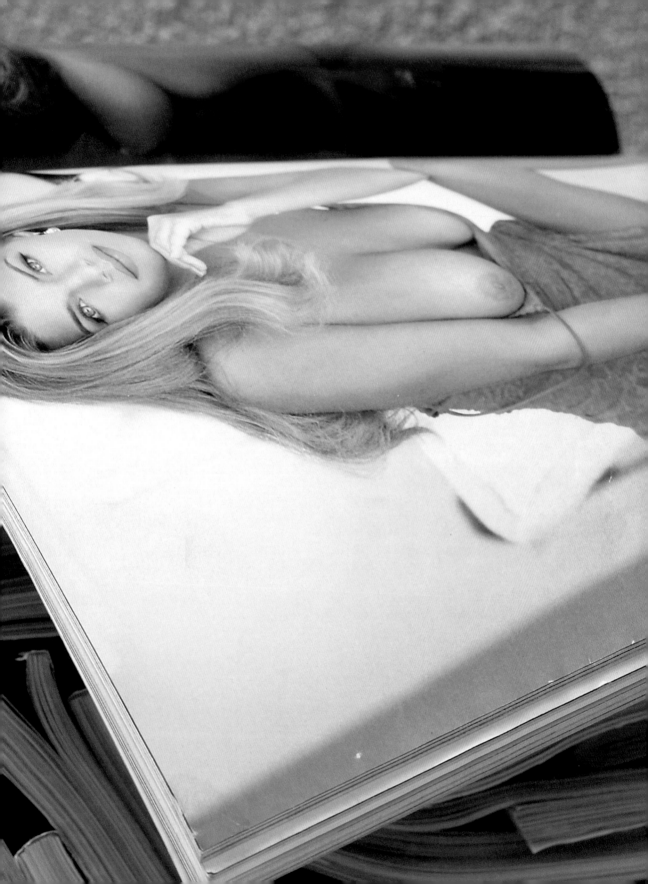

How much is too much?

Porn is there to jazz things up, not to replace real sex so watch just enough. It's there to make you want sex, want more sex, give you ideas and make you feel "naughty." If you find your usual bread-and-butter romp uninspiring and unappealing after watching porn, tone down the porn or up the ante in your real-life bedroom.

Keep it real
Some men say a steady diet of porn does leave them desensitized and one, lone, imperfect girlfriend in the bed can seem a bit lacking. "It's easy to fix, though," says one of my porn-enthusiast male friends—"You just close your eyes and pretend she's the porn chick." Yup, that would work. But at some point you *do* have to open your eyes and it'd be nice for both of you if you didn't think "Oh, it's you" when you see it's just Jane on the end of your penis. If perfect porn chicky-babes are the *only* girls you watch and fantasize about, it will interfere with real-life sex. Enforce a porn ban for a while or watch amateur porn, where the bodies are more real.

Mix it up
Vary the porn so you don't become "addicted" to a certain type. If you're constantly tuned into Big Busty Babes, your girlfriend's B cup isn't going to do it for you. And it's easy to become used to certain stimuli— especially if it's effective. But just as it's unhealthy to *only* be able to orgasm using a vibrator or by having oral sex, it's unhealthy to watch the same type of porn. Mix it up a bit—and a *lot* with real sex. Especially if you're a guy. If you frequently masturbate to porn, you'll train yourself to orgasm quickly, and forget what foreplay even is.

I don't know anyone who's ever watched a porn movie all the way through because they're usually so badly acted and scripted, but you could give it a try!

What to do during it

Don't be surprised if you giggle nervously or laugh hysterically when you first turn it on. You're nervous—and a lot of porn is *sooooo* bad, it's funny. But even if that atrociously acted scenario is about as likely to happen in real life as I have winning the lottery without a ticket, it is sexy watching other people have sex. In between the laughter, try any or all of the following:

- Start watching the movie to get in the mood and then just leave it playing in the background as you get down to business. Glance up now and again to keep things nicely revved up.

- Take turns to watch—you give him oral while he enjoys the film, then he returns the favor.

- Use it to test out or learn how to do something you and your partner would both like to try. (Just be aware the people on screen are different than the norm. As in able to do stuff we can't and probably don't want to!)

- Use it to get ideas for sex positions to copy.

- Get into sex positions where you can both watch. Reverse cowgirl (her on top but facing away from him) or him-from-behind as you spoon, facing the TV. Doggie style also works well.

- Use your hands on each other while your eyes are trained on the screen.

- Tie your partner up, then put the movie on. Masturbate in front of them but don't touch them.

- Tie your partner up, put the film on, and then tease them mercilessly before having your wicked way. Next time, they do it to you.

- Blindfold them so they can hear but not see, as you describe what's happening and act it out.

- Watch the whole thing and have sex afterward, roleplaying what you've just seen.

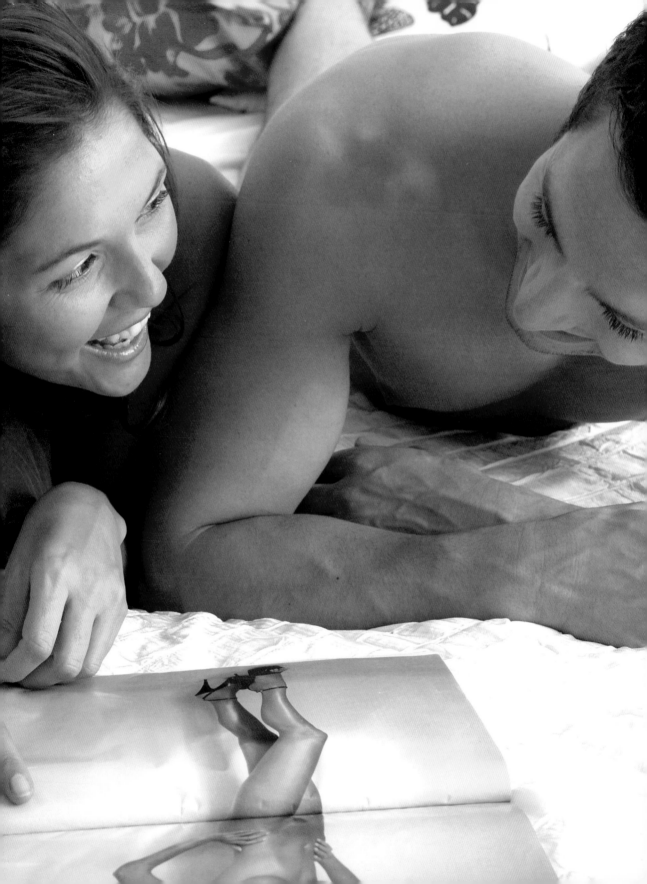

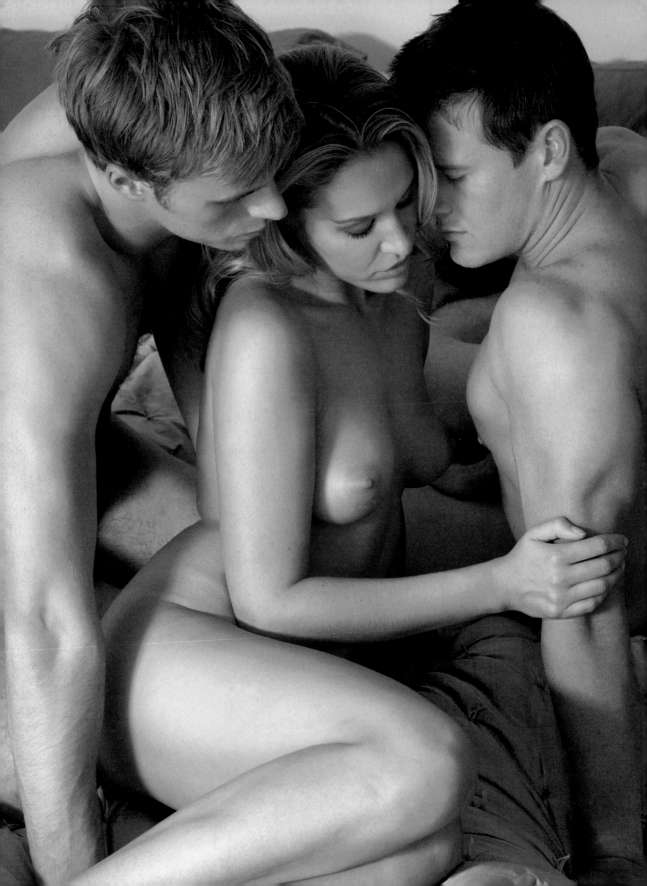

How To Have A Threesome

It's twice the stimulation so surely twice the fun, right? Hmm. I'm not convinced but if you're intent on having a threesome, at least do it the right way. Here are some practical guidelines for those who do want to try group sex without getting hurt ...

Here's a shocking fact: I've never had a threesome. Yep. Me! For some reason people find this truly astonishing (assuming, I think, that because I write about sex, I'll have done *everything*). Why haven't I had one? Well, when I would have been up for it (young, stoned, in college, not in love), I was too thick to pick up on all those veiled suggestions that were made.

Like the time I stayed at a friend's house who I hadn't seen since school. She made up the spare bed (a thin, lumpy mattress on the floor in the living room, one threadbare sheet), then took me up to her bedroom to show me the big, comfy, inviting king-size bed she shared with her boyfriend. He was already in it. "Are you sure you wouldn't be more comfortable in here?" she said with a smile. Considering this was the same girl who used to get her previous boyfriend to kiss me when we were drunk to "see what I kissed like," how could I miss what she really meant? But I did. "I couldn't possibly make you and your boyfriend sleep on the floor," I said. At which point she rolled her eyes at the ceiling and her boyfriend and gave up, clearly deciding if I was that stupid, I'd be lousy in bed anyway. (This is nothing new, by the way: I totally missed the whole coke thing as well because I could never work out who the hell "charlie" was and didn't want to ask because clearly everyone knew, apart from me.)

By the time I did get the message—i.e. "I can't believe you haven't had a threesome! Want one with us?" ultra-obvious offers—I was either in a relationship or knew myself too well. I'm way, way too jealous to share, plus I sort of think I've missed the boat. Threesomes tend to work best when you're young, not in a relationship, and partying your ass off. It's not that I'm staying in knitting, I just know too much about what can go wrong.

So who am I to tell you how to have one? Well, through research, including information from sex therapists, psychologists, and anyone else I thought could offer a useful opinion, and interviewing people who've had first-hand experience. Can I just say, I don't think a threesome is going to be the best idea you've had. Possibly it's the worst. So I am NOT recommending them. I simply know there are some people reading this book who will have one regardless of the risks and if you're intent on doing it, I'm equally as determined to make sure you do it in the least harmful way possible.

Try talking about threesomes to friends and see if anyone suddenly drops by asking for a cup of sugar at 11pm on a Saturday night.

1

The main attraction is you're the center of attention, and if you're bored with your sex life, it's something deliciously taboo for you to do!

2

Some feel it's instructive to watch other people's sexual techniques, others that it's a more honest way to sleep with other people.

3

Some believe there's no such thing as fidelity and it's better to let a partner indulge an urge in front of you so you feel involved and in control.

4

Group sex is all about instant gratification and it's far less personal than one-on-one. If you're after emotionless sex, it's perfect.

Why it can go horribly, horribly wrong ...

The obvious, most glaring reason is that couples that love each other usually have a hard time seeing their partners with someone else. Most of us are pretty territorial about relationships and our partners, and are not used to sharing them. No matter how much you've imagined it, you can't really prepare yourself for what it feels like to watch someone else kiss/touch/cuddle/lick/shag your partner.

– **The fantasy and reality don't match.** Things always go a lot smoother in our heads than they do in the bed.

– **It's awkward.** No one knows who's supposed to do what to who or when. Polite couples can find it turns into a "No, you go," "No, no, *you* go." Meanwhile the third person's rolling their eyes and examining their nails.

– **You both feel horribly self-conscious as well.** Sure, you've made love with your partner before but not had them *watch* you from a distance. And what if the third person thinks that killer blow-job your partner loves

is lousy? Will he then also think you're bad in bed? Performance anxiety is common for both men and women—especially if you're not terribly experienced.

– **Most of us cast ourselves** in the taking role when we imagine having a threesome, and get a bit put out when we realize this isn't necessarily the case.

– **Men often feel under so much pressure** to perform with two women, they can't get an erection. His sexual confidence is shattered to smithereens (What the hell does he tell the guys?) and the ramifications can be dire. The best way to ensure impotence isn't recurring is for men to forget about the time they had a one-off problem. Pretty hard to forget about this one.

– **Men often fare worse.** Lesbians consistently rate highest for the group most happy with their sex life. Watching your wife have more and better orgasms with a woman than she's ever had with you is another nail in the coffin of sexual confidence.

– **If it's a MMF combo,** watching your boyfriend or husband interact with another man can also be quite a shock. In your fantasy, both the men focus on *you*

that's sort of the point, after all). One friend told me, "I watched my man's hand reach over to grab the other guy's penis and then lean forward for a kiss and I was so shocked it made me feel a bit sick." Don't know about you, but I've never found throwing up in bed terribly sexy. Even if you can handle it, it's normal for thoughts of "Is he bi-curious or secretly gay?" to plague you afterward.

Lots of people end up in a threesome drunk, stoned, or high on drugs like E or Coke and do it because it seemed like such a good idea at the time. All these work wonders to reduce inhibitions. Trouble is your judgement—crucial in situations like this – disappears faster than your clothes. The ability to "read" your partner—who may be less into it than you are—is fatally flawed. Sometimes people keep going out of sheer "politeness" or because they think their partner's enjoying it and might get annoyed if they stop. You need one eye focused on your partner the entire time—especially if it's your first time—to check they really are fine. If you're seeing six in the bed and having trouble focusing on anything, you're in trouble.

Someone always gets blamed if the experience wasn't great. Even if you both came up with the idea together (which rarely happens), it's a natural human instinct to want to take it out on someone. This might be yourself or your partner. Either way, not huge fun.

People say the "trust bond" is broken, even if you've both agreed on it. If the threesome was with someone you know, any future contact could now been seen as a desire for a repeat performance, or that your partner's secretly fallen for the other person and wants to leave you for them. Some people *do* fall in love with the third party and ditch their partner. It doesn't happen often but it can, particularly if the person is a friend.

It can leave a bad feeling. Lots of people feel guilty, cheap, or disgusted with themselves afterward. Sometimes those feelings kick in *during* the threesome: once you've had an orgasm, the feeling can very quickly change from sexy to sordid.

Post-threesome blues also hit the third person in the bed. It's common to feel flat and lonely afterward. The couple snuggle in, you're pushed out.

Three's a crowd

Jealousy is an enormous problem—there's three of you in the bed remember, not two or four, so one person will sometimes feel left out and left thinking:

– Do they fancy the new person more than me? Are they enjoying themselves more with them than they do with me?

– Is this person better in bed and acting like your partner's the best thing in bed since the vibrator?

– Catch a glimpse of chemistry between the two of them that's missing in your relationship and suddenly it's not half as much fun. Lots of people are well aware of this and are inhibited for fear of upsetting their partner. And if you can't let loose and enjoy yourself, what's the point?

But for some, having more than one person want you, even fight over you, is an ego boost. Some find jealousy adds zing to tired relationships—others find it arousing to see someone else make love to their partner. It makes them feel desirable, being with someone who is desired.

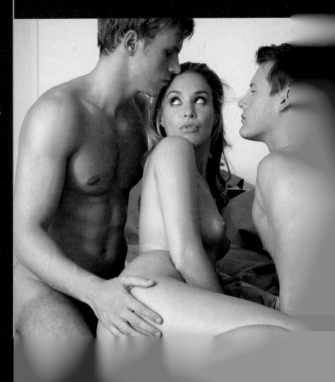

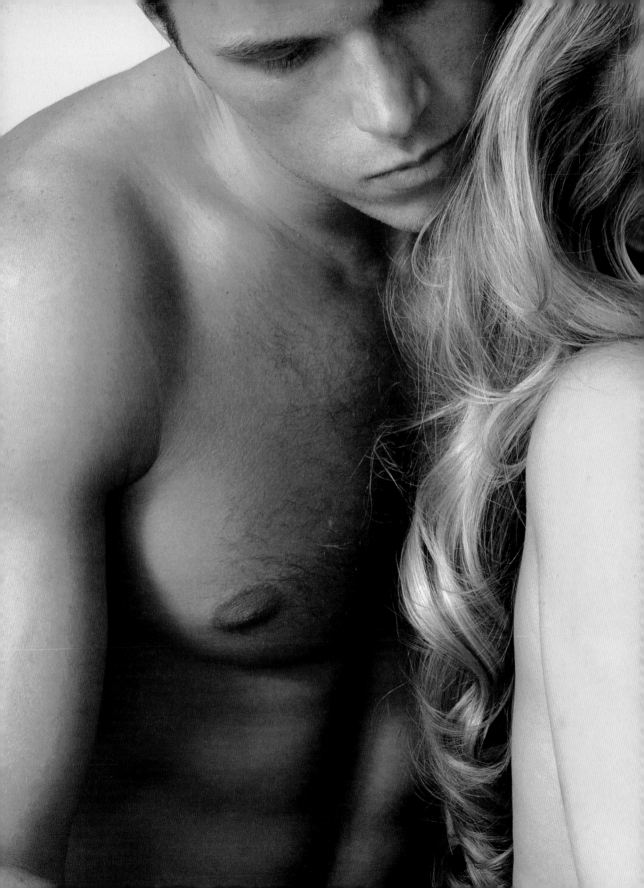

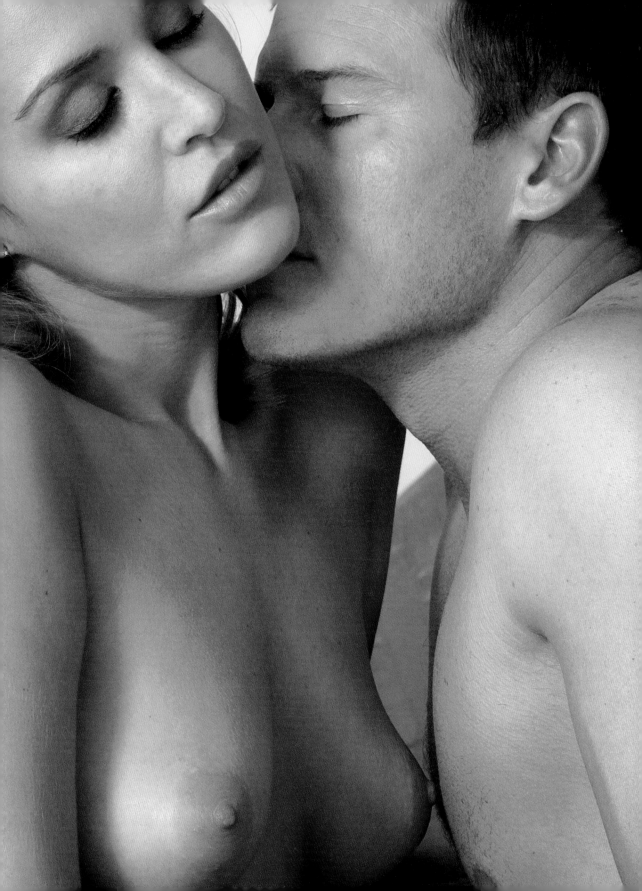

Who survives a threesome?

Most people don't but some can handle it ...

– Gay guys don't survive, they thrive! Just about every (handsome) gay friend of mine who isn't in a serious relationship seems to have at least two threesomes a month. Men clearly are better at separating sex from emotion. A fair few also don't have problems with threesomes even when in a committed relationship. (In the next life, I am coming back as a handsome gay man.)

– Singles who sleep with couples or people they don't know and will never see again. Even better if none of the three of you are involved with each other. This is the least risky situation to be in.

– Couples who aren't exclusive and like rather than love each other.

– Couples who are able to handle a one-off "treat." One couple I know hired a sex worker abroad and said it made for great fantasy material.

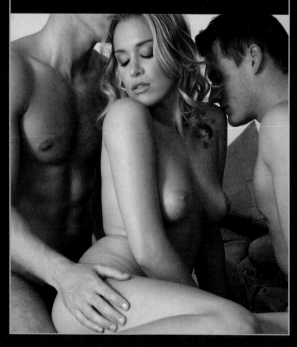

How to do it

Find someone to do it with
First up, you need to decide what combo you want—two men and one woman, two women and one man, three men, three women. Sexual preference obviously plays a part but always check the combination before you agree. (Again obvious but I've heard of a few jaws dropping when someone of the wrong sex arrives!)

Where to find a threesome
You could try talking about threesomes to friends and see if anyone suddenly drops by for a cup of sugar at 11pm on a Saturday night. Just be warned sleeping with friends is by far the riskiest option. The safest option if you're a couple is to hire a sex worker and meet them at a hotel—anonymity, little risk of a relationship developing, everyone knows what they're there for, and less obligation to keep going if you decide it's not for you. Just pay her or him and leave. Even better, do all this while you're abroad.

On the net, you'll find like-minded people in chatrooms, or Google "sex party" or "swinging" and you'll find no end of venues. I'm not saying you'll want to shag (or even talk) to all these people, but they will want what you want. The other option is to place or answer an ad.

Playing it safe
Some (sensible and more exclusive) clubs will ask you to provide proof you're HIV negative. There are also "safe sex parties" where everyone wears condoms and uses latex dams etc. Perhaps not surprisingly, these can be difficult to find. Always remember, condoms aren't absolute protection against STIs. Fingers, tongues, semen, skin-to-skin contact—all spread infection. (The only way to guarantee you won't catch something is to go along to a swingers' club and get your kicks simply by watching.) Change condoms between partners and positions, by the way.

If you've met online or through an advertisement, it's prudent to all meet beforehand and not give out personal details until then. Not just to check you fancy each other but to check they're not complete crazies. Trust your instincts. If you sense there is something weird (in a bad way), don't go there. I'd still consider meeting in a hotel rather than inviting them to your home.

Polite couples can find it turns into a "No, you go first," "No, no, *you* go." Meanwhile the third person's rolling their eyes and examining their nails.

Lots of people use drugs before or during a threesome. Only do this if you know the people you're sleeping with. Even then, please God tell me you've got the sense not to do them the first time around so you've got a hope of surviving emotionally. It's also advisable not to do too many drugs if you want to remember anything after.

Set the rules
Read all the negatives I've so subtly placed before you so you know what can go wrong. Most importantly, talk through *everything*: What if one person wants to stop and the other doesn't? (Come up with a code word that means "stop.") What if you want to do it again with the same person? (This is when emotions start getting involved.) What's allowed? Kissing, oral, intercourse, anal? Who's having sex with who? Are there any combinations that are banned/desired? Stick to the rules. Your relationship is always more important than the sex.

What to do while you're there
In some threesomes one person makes love to someone else while the other watches. (Common with couples where she wants to sleep with women and he's happy to indulge her if he can watch.) Another option is to "pair off" while one watches, then you swap. The usual is to try to make sure all three play at the same time by making a chain—he's licking her, she's being licked and also fellating the third guy, for instance. Make sure you balance the give-take ratio. If there's one final piece of advice it's this: *always* make your partner the "star" of the show and never, ever the other person. Unless you *want* to spend the next 20 years facing the same accusation—"You so fancied them more than me!"— over and over and over ... you get the picture. *For advice on how to suggest a threesome, see page 117.*

Who doesn't survive a threesome?

... and some can't.

– Couples who are in love and find the reality of sharing too hard to cope with.

– Couples where one partner feels pressured or there are threats: "If you won't do it, someone else will" or "I'll leave you if you don't do it."

– When one partner's agreed to the threesome just because the other wants to.

– When either of you are jealous, sexually insecure, or have body or trust issues.

– Couples who haven't thought through all possible scenarios properly. There should be no surprises.

– Older, long-term couples. It nearly always turns into an emotional disaster in this case because there's usually some unresolved sexual baggage just waiting to be reignited in a situation like this.

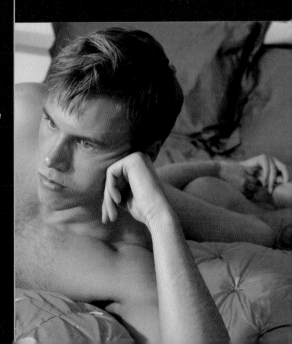

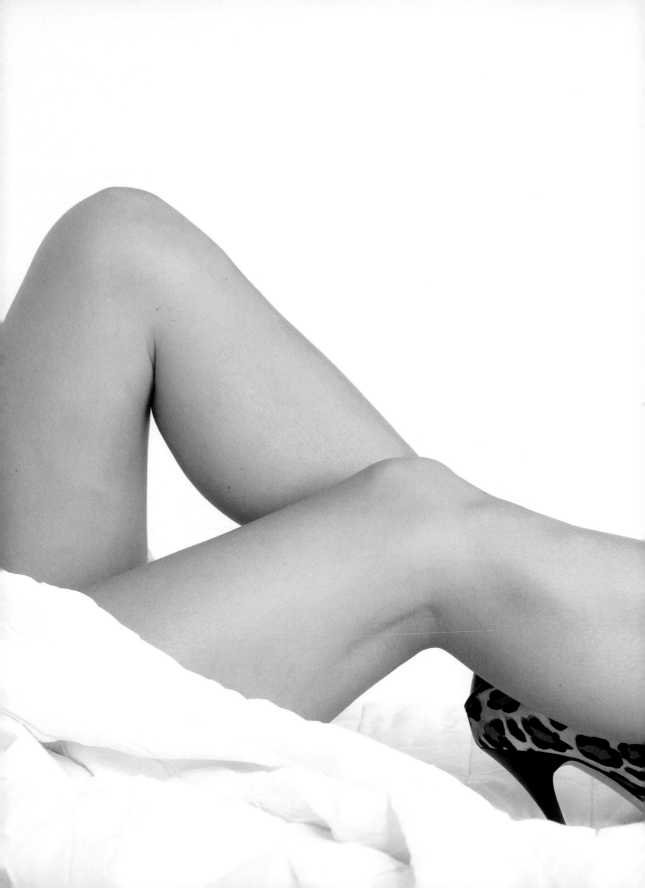

Chapter Five
Believing It

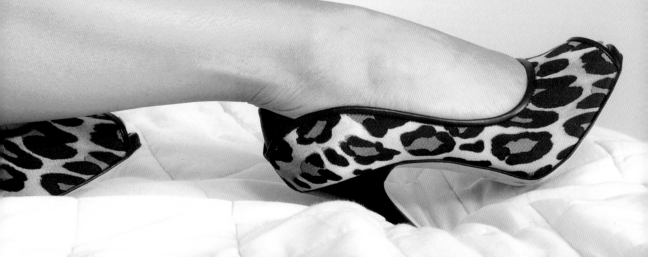

Sex Stuff That's Seriously Odd

Virgins who catch salmon with their bare hands, men who have sex with trash bags, the woman who has 200 orgasms a day … welcome to the weird and wacky world of fascinating, freakish sex.

This is, without apology, not going to improve your sex life in the slightest. I've written it purely for the amusement and fascination factor, as a salute to how diverse—and perverse—human sexuality really is.

Ancient weird stuff

You might get a "purity ring" and a pat on the head by an abstinence group for preserving your virginity today, but it was revered by ancient (and not so ancient) cultures. Each developed its own method of authenticating virgins. The Incas in South America believed the breath of a virgin could ignite a smoldering fire. (An evil non-virgin was brought in to put the fire out.) In the Jewish Talmud, you would straddle an open wine cask while a rabbi smelled your breath. If you'd done the deed, the wine fumes would have a clear path upward.

Meanwhile, in ancient China, there was the "pigeon egg test": the small, delicate egg would be pressed against the vagina and if it could be pushed inside, you'd failed the test dismally. Dismal being an understatement since virginity was so sacred back then, committing suicide was seen as the only way out if you succumbed too early. "Chastity arches" were provided for young girls who'd voluntarily hang themselves to restore the family's good name. In medieval Europe, virgins were blessed with magic powers: able to pass through fires without burning, hold poisonous snakes without being bitten, and catch salmon in their bare hands.

Modern-day weird stuff

Back on present-day Planet Earth, you'd think we'd have sorted our lives out a little by now. But no, we're still just as crazy as we ever were. There are so many bizarre stories of sexual behavior to choose from, it killed me to narrow it down to these little gems.

- **There's the Englishman** jailed first for having sex with the pavement in 1993, then two years later for doing it in public with a trash bag.

- **The Belgian optician** who, in 1995, was arrested for making his female patients strip and dance to accordian music before he'd fit their contact lenses.

- **The Pennsylvania judge** who, in 1992, promised to let criminals off if they let him shampoo their hair.

- **The US man** who, in 1992, was arrested for shooting himself repeatedly for sexual kicks while wearing a bullet-proof vest.

- **The proud Frenchman** who left his 9¾ in- (25 cm-) penis to a friend in his will.

- **A 1948 survey** found 8 percent of adult US males had enjoyed sexual contact with animals, and it seems we're still quite fond of it. In 1998, a man in San Francisco was charged with running a sex dungeon where you could have sex with an anteater, eels, and water buffalo.

What the hell is that?

Here's a glossary for those of you who want to understand porn jargon that's a little more hardcore. Be warned: some of this stuff is very out there, and some of it is downright dangerous. Do not try this at home!

AC/DC
A bisexual man.

ATM
"Ass to mouth" as in a finger, penis, or sex toy inserted up someone's bottom then popped right into a mouth. Can cause potentially life-threatening diseases.

Autoerotic asphyxiation
The act of choking someone until they almost die in order to intensify orgasm. Can go fatally wrong.

Back spackle
Ejaculating on someone's back or bottom.

CBT
Cock and ball torture. It can cause irreparable damage.

Cream pie
A woman with semen dripping from her anus or vagina.

DA
Double anal: two penises in one bottom (yes, it's possible).

DP
Double penetration: in the vagina and in the bottom.

Edge play
Sex involving injury, death, or humiliation. Do yourself a favor, don't go there.

Feature
Porn with a plot.

Felching
Sucking fluids from the vagina or anus. Poses the same health risks as ATM.

Fingercuffing
Being penetrated while sucking another man.

Fisting
Inserting a whole hand into the vagina or anus.

Fluffer
Someone who gives oral or hand-jobs to male porn stars before they go on camera. These days it tends to be DIY.

Gape or gaping
A vagina or anus stretched or held open to create a hole.

Glory hole
A hole in the wall that someone inserts a penis into anonymously, while someone on the other side sucks it.

Golden shower
The act of peeing on others or being peed on.

Money shot/Pop shot
Ejaculating for the camera. The longer the semen spurts out and the more of it there is, the better.

Pearl necklace
Ejaculating on to a women's neck and breasts so that the semen looks like a necklace.

Pony boy/girl
A male or female who pretends to be a pony in a submissive roleplay game. Some wear a saddle.

Pro-am
A professional amateur—meaning some of the "stars" are "real people" as opposed to porn stars.

Raincoater
The industry term for someone who buys porn films.

Tea-bagging
Dipping testes on to someone's face or into their mouth.

Wall-to-wall
One sex act after another without even a pretense of plot. Possibly the most honest porn flick of all.

Watersports
Being aroused by peeing on someone or being peed on.

AC/DC

ATM

Autoerotic

Asphyxiation

Back spackle

Bondage

CBT

Cream pie

DA

Dildo

DP

Edge play

Feature

Felching

Fingercuffing

Fisting

Fluffer

Gape or gaping

Glory hole

Golden shower

Money shot

Nipple clamp

Pearl necklace

Pony boy/girl

Pro-am

Raincoater

S&M

Speciality porn

Strap on

Teabagging

Wall to wall

Watersports

1

A man who injected cocaine into his penis ended up with gangrene and it fell off in the tub. He also lost both his legs and nine fingers.

2

In 1999, a blond porn star called Houston decided to hold the World's Biggest Gangbang, getting through exactly 620 men in one session.

3

A teacup, a pair of glasses, a frozen pig's tail, a flashlight, and a jar of peanut butter have been removed by doctors from the male rectum.

4

Dr. John Harvey Kellogg invented breakfast cereal as an antidote to masturbation. He believed sex was "injurious to health."

– **Not only are we having sexual contact** with animals, we're also getting caught. One can only imagine the humiliation felt by the 59-year-old man from Sussex, England, who, in 1994, sat his friends down to watch a wedding video, inserted the wrong tape, and instead treated them to a video of him having sex with the neighbor's dog. It's uncertain whether the neighbors were there at the time, but you can bet Rover was kept inside from then on.

– **Sweet but somewhat misguided** was the 85-year-old Sicilian man who stabbed his wife in the shoulder when he found a hot, passionate letter addressed to her. It turned out to be written by him, 50 years earlier.

Just plain weird
"Everyone to his own taste and mine is for corpses," said Henry Blot, a famous necrophiliac at his trial in the 19th century. He'd continued to have sex with his wife for seven years after her death. If you think that's odd, cast a suspicious eye over anyone abnormally absorbed in the Statue of David. A galateist or agalmatophiliac is a person sexually attracted to statues or mannequins.

People, mainly men, who join "Diaper Clubs" suffer from anaclitism: needing to wear or use objects usually used by infants—pacifiers, diapers, rattles—before they can become aroused. Less common but difficult if you're a churchgoer or public speaker is being a homilophiliac: someone who becomes sexually aroused while listening to or giving sermons or speeches. Interestingly, this can be traced back to ancient religious services that were in fact designed to arouse devotees sexually in preparation for the orgies that followed. In modern times, it's thought guilt plays a big part in producing this passionate response: if someone's lecturing passionately against the sins of sex, it can cause the audience to be more aroused than if they were watching porn. Anything forbidden becomes intensely desirable.

On a more lighthearted note—though in reality, it's apparently exhausting—is the story of Sarah Carmen from the UK who has 200 orgasms per day due to Permanent Sexual Arousal Syndrome (PSAS). This condition, also called Persistent Genital Arousal Disorder, increases blood flow to the genitals and results in spontaneous and constant arousal, often unrelated to sexual desire. It can be set off by the mere rumble of a distant train or the vibrations of a hairdryer.

Some of this research was drawn from the following books: Sex, A User's Guide by Stephen Arnott, The Book of Weird Sex *by Chris Gordon, and* The Encyclopedia of Unusual Sex Practices *by Brenda Love.*

5

In Victorian times, boys were stopped from masturbating by having their foreskin drawn forward, holes drilled through it, and lock and key laced through.

6

In Japan, there was a trade in used panties of schoolgirls, housewives, nurses, and widows. You could also buy bottles of schoolgirl saliva.

In the eye of the beholder

Adolfus Frederick, King of Sweden (1751–1771) had seven mistresses: two were one-armed, two one-legged, two one-eyed, and one had no arms. He's thought to have been an acrotomophiliac: someone who has an erotic fixation with amputees. (You think?)

Because you can ...

If a man claims to be an autopederast, show respect. This means he's able to insert his own penis into his own anus. While it's not physically possible for most men, with a semi-erect penis, some achieve it.

Off with his penis!

Castration—removal of the testicles and/or penis—might be illegal today, but in times gone by, it was as common as a Roman orgy.

- The testicles were removed by either crushing, twisting, or tying a tight string around the scrotum, cutting off the blood supply and waiting till the whole thing dropped off. (I can see you wince from here.) If you were lucky, they simply used a knife. Why do it? Castrated men—eunuchs—were hotly pursued by royalty because they were considered to be good employees. Unambitious, loyal, and … yeah right, what everyone really meant was eunuchs were unlikely or unable to shag your wife or mistress.

- In Greece, eunuchs were employed to guard the King's harem; The Persian Emperor Darius (5th Century BC) was supplied with 500 castrated boys every year for employment within the palace. He liked them because they were "docile." Problem was, some took "docile" to the extreme and actually died. Around 90 percent, in fact, if both the penis and testicles were removed.

- If penises weren't being lopped off to create subservient men, warriors were cutting them off as battle trophies. The Hebrews liked snipping off their enemies' foreskins as war mementos (sentimental folk that they were); the ancient Egyptians and Ethiopians went the whole nine yards and took the penis, too. Pharaoh Menephta collected 13,240 penises from dead Libyan soldiers in 1300 BC to celebrate his victory.

- In more recent times, a housewife in China decided to "prune" her underperforming husband. She cut off his penis thinking it might grow back bigger and stronger. It didn't. There's also the infamous story of two Thai wives who made damn sure their husbands' cut-off penises couldn't be reattached. One, rather ingeniously, tied her husband's severed member to a helium balloon, the other chucked it out the window—straight into the mouth of a duck.

What The Hell Do I Do Now?

Not wanting to look sexually stupid or cast our lovers in a bad light, plenty of people keep quiet about potentially embarrassing sex situations, preferring to suffer in dignified silence. Silly when most are remarkably easy to fix …

Some sex problems we'll cheerfully blab to friends about after a few wines because we secretly think they make us look good. The old "He's too big for me," for instance. Confessing this problem not only lets our girlfriends know the new guy's hung like a horse, it also craftily implies we're as tight as a virgin. We're not quite as quick to confess things that don't paint such a complimentary picture—like him not getting hard enough or not fancying sex at all—and we're particularly reluctant to talk about things that might suggest we're not as sexually savvy as we like to make out. Instant Sex Makeovers (see pages 116–123) provided quick fix-its to common sex dilemmas, here you'll find solutions to things that are a little more delicate to handle, along with answers to questions you might be embarrassed to ask because they just seem way too obvious.

What to do when …

A sex toy gets lost
And I'm not talking about wondering which drawer you left it in or losing it under the bed. If you've been a little over-enthusiastic, condoms, dildos, vibrators, or butt plugs can disappear out of reach inside rectums or vaginas. Out of the two, it's less of a problem if something's lodged high in the vagina because there's an "end" to it. Chances are the pesky little condom or love egg is hiding above or behind the cervix. To get to it, simply fish around with your fingers until you find something that feels like the top of your nose and hook your fingers around to feel in the nook behind it.

Losing something up your bottom is more of a worry because the object can move upward into the large intestine. This is why anal toys have flared bases, to stop you from inserting it so far the toy suddenly decides to pack a lunch and set off exploring on its own. It's hard not to panic if this does happen, but the best thing to do is simply to wait for your next bowel movement and see if it makes a reappearance. If it doesn't, or you experience any sort of fever, abdominal pain, or start to bleed, I'm afraid it's off to the emergency room *immediately*. And yes, it will be embarrassing but believe me, they've seen far worse than this.

You don't know how to use a vibrator
It might sound obvious but read the instructions. Try the different settings, get a feel of where the switches are, experiment with the different levels of vibration, then grab your usual masturbation turn-on—a book, your laptop for some online porn, or start running a well-worn "taped" fantasy in your head. Get into position—and take your pick. Depending on the vibrator, you can squat over it, lie back and hold it between your legs, clamp it there with your thighs, or lie on your tummy and do the same. Hold it over your clitoris and alter the speed, pressure, and angle until it starts to feel good. If it feels too intense, put a T-shirt between it and you. Try angling

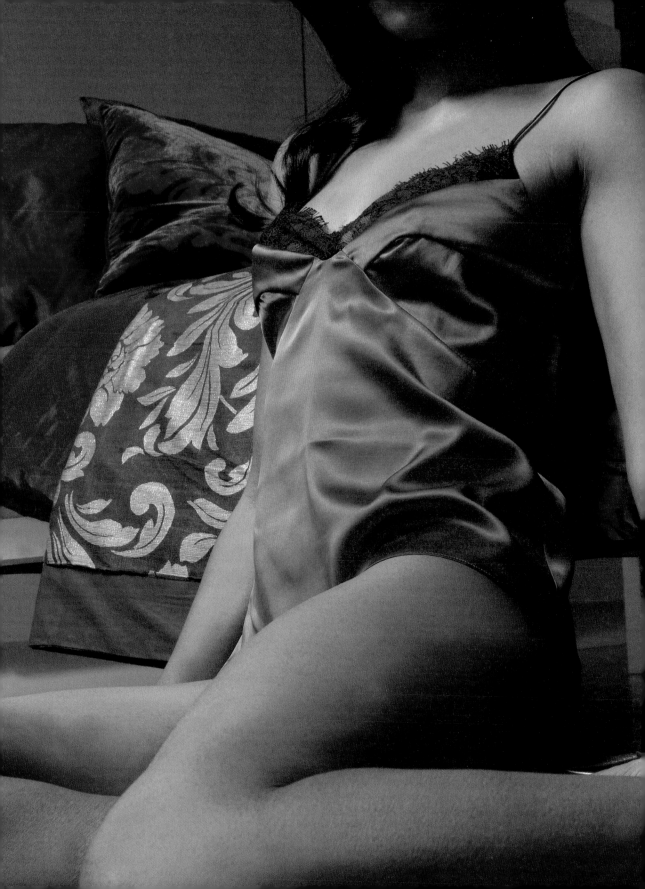

What to do if he falls out all the time

This may be happening because you've used too much lube or you're very wet—both problems are easily fixed by using a small towel to wipe away the excess. The position, size of his penis, and thrusting style are also factors. If his penis is quite short and he thrusts long—pulling back on each stroke rather than staying deep inside you—it's bound to happen. The bigger he is and the closer he holds you, the less likely he is to fall out. But there are also ways you can help:

- Hold him close by grabbing on to his buttock cheeks or wrapping your legs tightly around him when he's inside you.

- Reach around with your hand and hold onto the base of his penis to keep him inside.

- When choosing your position, bear in mind your vagina curves up toward your tummy. Does his erection point a particular way? Most point up but some stick straight out or point downward.

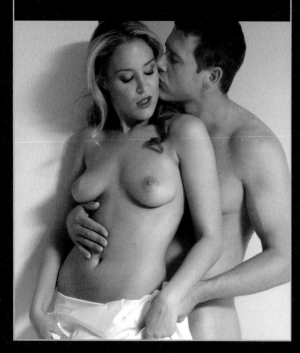

it so it's jutting into the side of the clitoris, with the outer labia as a buffer. Adjust the intensity by putting your hand over it to absorb the vibration, remove it when you want it stronger again. You could also try holding your middle fingers over your clitoris and putting the vibrator on top. Once you've got the hang of it—which should only take about five minutes—you'll be more than impressed with your new toy. It's for this reason I recommend you don't rely exclusively on it for your orgasms. Vibrators don't make mistakes, humans do. Tongues get tired, fingers fumble. And clitorises get lazy and refuse to play the orgasm game if you only ever play it one way. Try to throw in at least two out of five orgasms via tongue/fingers or (if you're lucky) through penetration.

She doesn't like intercourse
Despite intercourse being one of the least effective ways to make her orgasm, most women still thoroughly enjoy a good rogering—if it's done well. If you penetrate too quickly and launch into "the jackhammer", then given the choice between shagging you or filling in her tax return, she's going to get out the calculator every time. So first up, slow it down. Up the amount of foreplay beforehand and use lube if she's not wet enough. Experiment with different speeds, depths, angles, and rhythms of thrusting. Keep your pelvises close, put your hands on her butt cheeks, and hold her as close as you can, grinding in a circular fashion. Keep your eyes open to stay connected to her, kiss her mouth, and her neck. Offer clitoral stimulation of some sort—either use your fingers or buy a small classic cylindrical vibrator and put that on her clitoris while you're inside her. Don't go on thrusting forever but learn how to control yourself a little. Most women are happy with anything from five to 10 minutes of intercourse.

You're mismatched physically
He's six foot six and you're scraping five foot, one of you is way heavier than the other … love might conquer all but sex can be a literal pain if your body parts are completely disparate. The solution: find ways to even things up—use the stairs, pillows, or furniture designed expressly for this purpose. Anyone who's appreciated a well-placed pillow under the hips—for comfort or to alter sensation—will get the concept of sex furniture. We've all heard of sex swings but that's just the tip of the iceberg. "Wedges" are portable, firm, wedge-shaped

pillows you lie on or slide under your hips or bottom to prop up parts during intercourse or oral sex. "Ramps" put you at dramatic angles to reach parts you didn't even know existed. Sex furniture is ideal for couples who are mismatched physically but it's a hell of a lot of fun to use even if you aren't. Check out inflatable cushions, vibrating chairs, and sex sofas that range from inflatable and tacky to actually quite stylish chaise versions. Sex swings hang from the ceiling and can be quite an operation to install, but they can be effective if different weights are a problem.

You don't know how to use a dildo
Dildos (see pages 143–144) are useful if you're lesbian and don't have a penis handy for penetration, if you want penetration in more than one place but only have one penis to play with, or if he quite likes being penetrated anally. Dildos are way more versatile than the real thing because there's no body attached to that "penis." If you're experimenting solo, put some lube on you or the dildo, then go for it. If it comes with a suction cap, attach it at the appropriate level, then back on to it doggy style or crouch in "girl on top" position. Or lie on your back and use your hand to thrust it in and out, varying between long and deep and short and shallow strokes. Try playing with your clitoris at the same time or using a vibrator on it.

If you're using a dildo with your partner, try letting them insert a lubed-up dildo as they're giving you oral. (Vaginally or anally, if it's got a flared base.) Some women like it simply to be in there for pressure, others like it thrust in and out. If you fancy a threesome but don't want the emotional angst, this can feel like having two lovers at once. Get the same effect by him lying beside you kissing and playing with your breasts while he thrusts in and out with the dildo. (All these techniques also work with penetrative vibrators, by the way.)

He can't come through intercourse
First, let's give up the assumption that all guys can climax effortlessly, all the time, no matter what you dish up. Just as some women can only orgasm a particular way (most commonly through oral sex or with a vibrator) some guys are the same. His most reliable and frequent orgasms are nearly always DIY, by hand—his hand. If he's not climaxing easily through intercourse, it's often because he needs a specific stroke that he uses and

only a hand can provide. Your vagina (obviously) can't replicate firm, rhythmic tugging (kegel exercises work to a point but they're not *that* good). It could also be because he masturbates using a really hard grip—even the tightest vagina is no match for a firm fist. Get him to masturbate himself in front of you so you can see what technique he uses to make himself climax and how hard he holds himself. Then let him teach you how to replicate it. Hold him firmly around the base the next time he penetrates, and use your hand to slide up and down his penis as he slides up and down inside you, bearing in mind what stroke you know he likes. Tell him the firmer he grips himself during masturbation, the less likely he'll be to orgasm during intercourse with you. He can retrain his penis by using a lighter, gentler grip when he masturbates.

You can't stop fantasizing about someone
Like many people, you may have been guilty of playing out wicked little fantasies starring highly inappropriate people (your best friend's partner, your boss, your mother or father-in-law) in your head. Most of us, quite rightly, dismiss these mental erotic adventures as harmless or use them when we masturbate. Sometimes though, they can teeter on the edge of obsession, making you embarrassed, uncomfortable, and guilty whenever you're around the person. The way to stop it is to let yourself have the fantasy but give it a negative ending. You not only get caught in the act, you lose your partner, your home, your children, your friends, your reputation over it. The person you cheated with wants

Losing something up your bottom is more of a worry. This is why anal toys have flared bases—to stop you from inserting it in so far the toy suddenly decides to pack a lunch and set off exploring on its own.

His most reliable and frequent orgasms are nearly always DIY, by hand—his hand. Even the tightest vagina is no match for a firm fist.

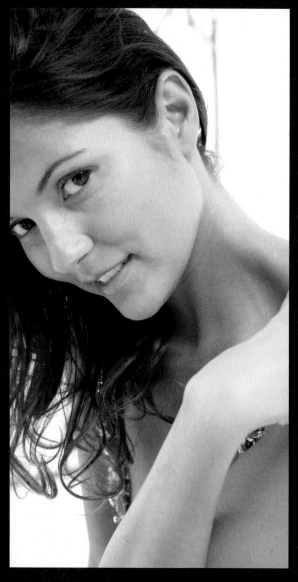

nothing to do with you, you're left alone and what for? Five minutes of satisfying a sexual itch. Do this each time the fantasy hits and I promise you your brain won't want to go there anymore.

She doesn't like you going down on her

A lot of the time it's because she's worried how she looks or tastes. You're getting a better view than she'll ever have unless she's held a hand mirror to see what's down there. Female genitals get a bad rap—if they're not "fishy," they're mushy and obviously smell because otherwise why would we need so many "feminine hygiene" products? It's no wonder lots of women are paranoid. The first thing to do is let her know how pretty she looks down there and how much it turns you on looking at her. Let her shower first if she's worried and make a big deal of telling her how much you like the way she tastes. Try putting a finger inside her and bringing it up to her nose and mouth, letting her smell and taste herself. This can allay some women's fears, but others may freak out (I'll let you be the judge of how your girlfriend is likely to react).

Compliments and reassurance should eventually do the trick, but if she's still reluctant after that it's likely to be because she's been brought up to believe genitals are "dirty" (strict parents or a religious background?) or perhaps she's had a bad experience in the past. Get her to try to open up about why she doesn't like it, but if she won't talk to you, suggest she reads some books for reassurance or visits a therapist for one or two sessions. Finally, what's your technique like? If you're too rough, she might be avoiding oral sex for that reason.

He's lost his erection

Women are timid around penises that aren't very hard. We'll grab on to it with gusto when it's solid and stiff but switch to a nervous, tentative touch the second there's any sign of softness. In fact, the opposite should happen. If he's only semi-erect, he'll usually appreciate a firm grip and firm massaging. Combine this with the right attitude—that it happens all the time and so isn't a big deal—and all will be solved. A soft penis is a lot easier to fellate because you can get the whole thing in there. It doesn't need to be fully erect to penetrate either—use your fingers to stuff it inside you and keep your hand down there to make sure it stays inside. Massage his testicles as he thrusts slow and steady to start with and if you can reach, firmly massage the perineum with the pads of your fingers. Above all, keep the pressure off and let him know you're completely unperturbed. If the relationship is new and your partner's had erection problems in the past, it could be he just needs time to feel completely comfortable with you.

She hates your hand-jobs

As a general rule, if she pulls away from your hand you're being too rough, if she pushes against it, you're being too gentle. If I had to place a bet though, I'd say the mistake you're making is the first one. The general consensus of what feels good for most women is to keep it gentle, soft, wet, and consistent. Next time, start by stroking her outer lips and letting them open naturally, then slowly slide a (wet or pre-lubed) finger between the lips of the inner labia. Don't hone in on the clitoris specifically until she's fully aroused, then try circling it with a fingertip before continuing with the sliding motion between the inner lips. Try dipping your fingers inside her vagina occasionally to keep things wet—also because penetration does feel good. (I know I've been knocking it but that's because I'm trying to get you to think outside the box.) Remember, the head is just the tip of the clitoris, stimulate the rest of it that's hidden below the surface using pressure and firm massage. As with oral sex, never change what you're doing once she's close to climaxing, though you might like to up the speed and pressure a little.

Some sex problems we'll cheerfully blab to friends about. The old "He's too big for me," for instance, lets our girlfriends know the new guy's hung like a horse, and it craftily implies we're as tight as a virgin.

Make condoms feel better

If he loses an erection when he pulls on a condom, it could be because it's too tight or too big—the first deadens sensation, the second friction. Experiment with different sizes and types but remember while there are condoms so thin you can't even feel them, the whole point of wearing one is for protection. Stick to reputable brands that have passed government safety standard tests and use lube *inside* the condom to make it feel better and provide maximum sensation for him; use a little more on the *outside* to reduce the risk of it tearing and to make it comfortable for her.

Make sure you use them correctly

Check the expiration date and don't rip the packet open with your teeth. Leave space at the tip for the semen to collect and withdraw quite quickly, before his erection completely subsides, with one of you holding on to the base of condom to stop it from slipping off. You won't be the first couple to look down in horror when you realize he's pulled his penis out but left the condom in there.

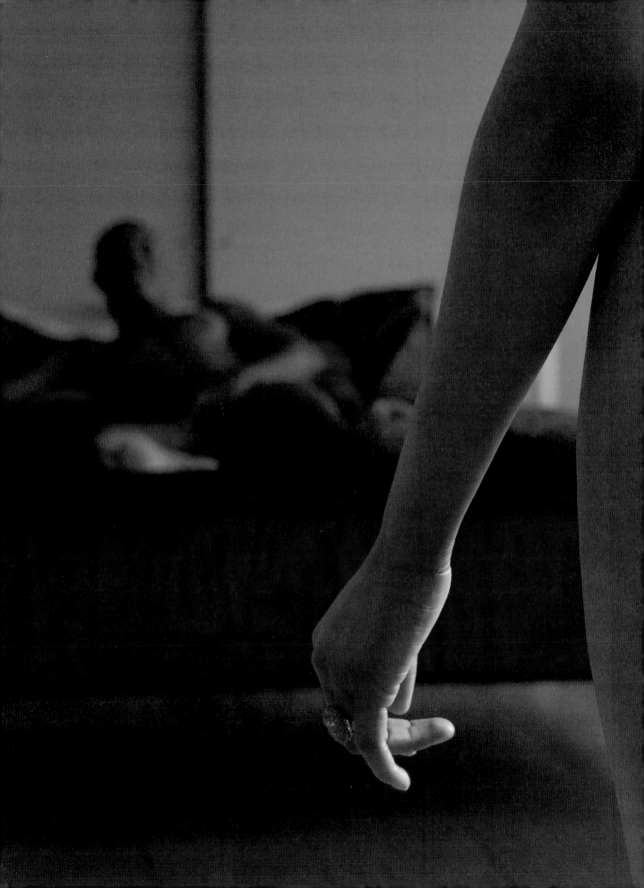

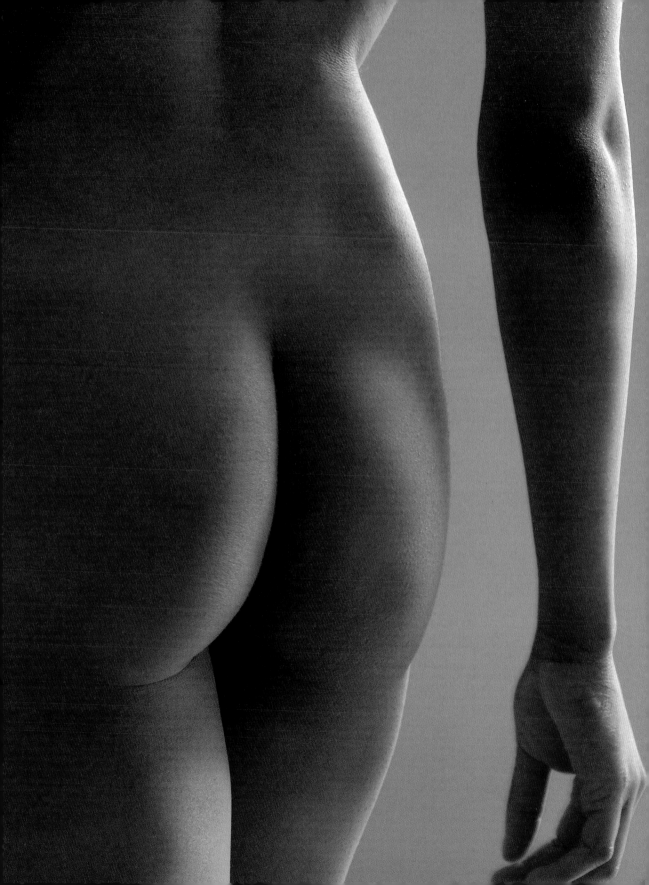

Index

Thanks

It is impossible to produce anything worthwhile without good friends, a supportive family, and talented colleagues and I was lucky enough to be blessed with all three while writing this book. An enormous thank you to all for being so patient, kind, and encouraging while I was invariably irritable, tense, and depressed, in the midst of deadline hell. While I'm certain all of you inwardly groan when I tell you I'm about to start writing another book, you never obviously wince and for that I'm grateful.

This is my 12th book and the first time I've had to adjust my list of family members to thank. This year has been tinged with a great deal of sadness because my mother's long-term partner Terry died suddenly. Quite simply, we miss him. My love for all my family is immense and very obvious to anyone who has seen us all together. Thanks to my mother Shirley, my father Patrick and his wife Maureen, my brother Nigel and his about-to-be-wife Diana, my sister Deborah and her husband Doug, and my beautiful niece and nephew, Maddie and Charlie. I hold you all in my heart in the hope of keeping you all safe.

Thanks also to Vicki McIvor, my agent and best friend. You never, ever fail to impress me with how hard you work, how little you complain, and how giving and loving you are with your time and your affection. Thank you also for sharing Lara, your daughter and my god-daughter. She is both outrageously entertaining and loveable and squeezes my heart every time she says "Aunty Tracey."

To all my closest, dearest friends for not giving me a hard time when I couldn't come out to play: Sandra Aldridge, Peggy Bunker, Rachel Corcoran, Claire Faragher, Catherine Jarvie, Karen Reid, Kate Morey, Steph Harris, Tracy Forsyth, Jeremy Milnes, and Fenella Thomas.

To my editor, Dawn Bates, for working ridiculously hard and long hours on this book and never once compromising your exceptionally high standards.

You are a joy to work with on every level and I honestly don't think I could have done it without you.

Thanks to Peter Jones at DK, as always, who casts a wise and shrewd eye over every sentence I write. You gave me encouragement when I needed it most and I appreciated it more than you could ever know.

To SEA, the design team behind this book and the photographer Andrew G. Hobbs. Thank you for lending a fresh, distinctive new look and for being patient with my (possibly relentless) demands. The end result is stunning and thanks, especially, to Ryan Jones and Lynsey McCarthy. Thanks also on the design side to Kat Mead at DK. It was lovely to work with someone so dedicated and enthusiastic, not to mention a brilliant sense of humor and loads of fun.

Thanks also to Richard Longhurst and Neal Slateford at Love Honey, not just for providing toys for the shoot but for producing my fabulous sex toy range and being so utterly delightful and entertaining to work with.

Finally, thanks to all at Dorling Kindersley, world-wide, for being so lovely to work with. In the UK office, the effervescent Stephanie Jackson, John Roberts, Deborah Wright, Serena Stent, Hermione Ireland, Catherine Bell, Adèle Hayward, Helen Poultney, and Helen Spencer. In the US office, Gary June, Therese Burke, Tom Korman, and Rachel Kempster, and in Canada, Chris Houston and Loraine Taylor.

DK would like to thank Andrew G. Hobbs and John Ross for the photography, Andi Sisodia for proofreading, and Dr. Laurence Errington for indexing.

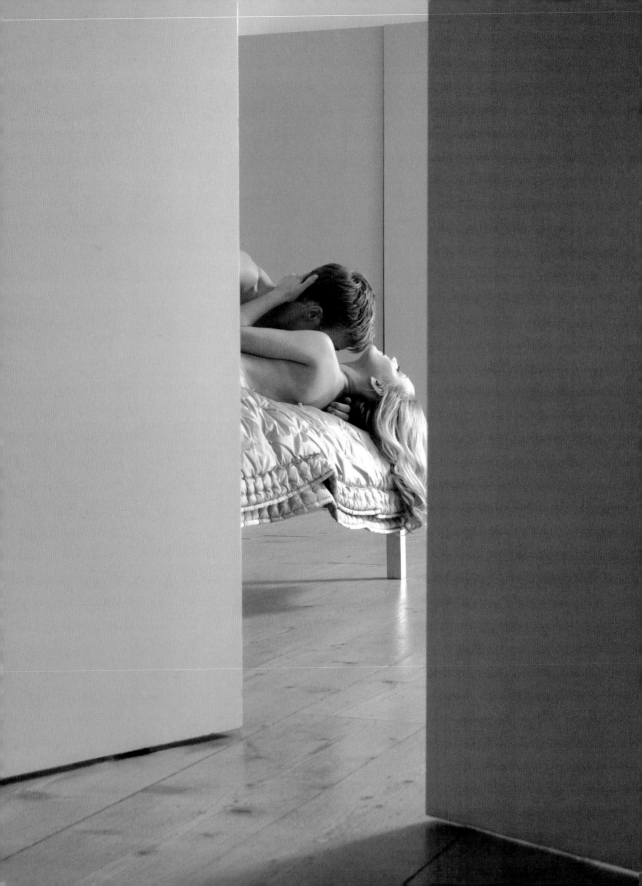